Lead Management for Electrophysiologists

Editors

NOEL G. BOYLE
BRUCE L. WILKOFF

CARDIAC ELECTROPHYSIOLOGY CLINICS

www.cardiacEP.theclinics.com

Consulting Editors
RANJAN K. THAKUR
ANDREA NATALE

December 2018 • Volume 10 • Number 4

ELSEVIER

1600 John F. Kennedy Boulevard • Suite 1800 • Philadelphia, Pennsylvania, 19103-2899

http://www.theclinics.com

CARDIAC ELECTROPHYSIOLOGY CLINICS Volume 10, Number 4
December 2018 ISSN 1877-9182, ISBN-13: 978-0-323-64101-2

Editor: Stacy Eastman
Developmental Editor: Donald Mumford

Cardiac Electrophysiology Clinics (ISSN 1877-9182) is published quarterly by Elsevier Inc., 360 Park Avenue South, New York, NY 10010-1710. Months of issue are March, June, September, and December. Subscription prices are $215.00 per year for US individuals, $344.00 per year for US institutions, $236.00 per year for Canadian individuals, $415.00 per year for Canadian institutions, $299.00 per year for international individuals, $415.00 per year for international institutions and $100.00 per year for US, Canadian and international students/residents. To receive student/resident rate, orders must be accompanied by name of affilliated institution, date of term, and the signature of program/residency coordinator on institution letterhead. Orders will be billed at individual rate until proof of status is received. Foreign air speed delivery is included in all Clinics subscription prices. All prices are subject to change without notice. **POSTMASTER:** Send address changes to Cardiac Electrophysiology Clinics, Elsevier Health Sciences Division, Subscription Customer Service, 3251 Riverport Lane, Maryland Heights, MO 63043. **Customer Service: 1-800-654-2452 (US and Canada). From outside of the US and Canada, call 314-477-8871. Fax: 314-447-8029. E-mail: JournalsCustomerService-usa@elsevier.com (for print support); JournalsOnlineSupport-usa@elsevier.com (for online support).**

Reprints. For copies of 100 or more of articles in this publication, please contact the Commercial Reprints Department, Elsevier Inc., 360 Park Avenue South, New York, NY 10010-1710. Tel.: 212-633-3874; Fax: 212-633-3820; E-mail: reprints@elsevier.com.

Cardiac Electrophysiology Clinics is covered in *MEDLINE/PubMed (Index Medicus).*

Contributors

CONSULTING EDITORS

RANJAN K. THAKUR, MD, MPH, MBA, FHRS
Professor of Medicine and Director, Arrhythmia Service, Thoracic and Cardiovascular Institute, Sparrow Health System, Michigan State University, Lansing, Michigan, USA

ANDREA NATALE, MD, FACC, FHRS
Executive Medical Director, Texas Cardiac Arrhythmia Institute, St. David's Medical Center, Austin, Texas; Consulting Professor, Division of Cardiology, Stanford University, Palo Alto, California; Adjunct Professor of Medicine, Heart and Vascular Center, Case Western Reserve University, Cleveland, Ohio; Director, Interventional Electrophysiology, Scripps Clinic, San Diego, California; Senior Clinical Director, EP Services, California Pacific Medical Center, San Francisco, California

EDITORS

NOEL G. BOYLE, MD, PhD, FHRS, FACC
Professor of Medicine, UCLA Cardiac Arrhythmia Center, David Geffen School of Medicine at UCLA, Ronald Reagan UCLA Medical Center, UCLA Health System, Los Angeles, California, USA

BRUCE L. WILKOFF, MD, FHRS, FACC, FAHA, CCDS
Professor of Medicine, Cleveland Clinic Lerner College of Medicine of Case Western Reserve University, Robert and Suzanne Tomsich Department of Cardiovascular Medicine, Director, Cardiac Pacing and Tachyarrhythmia Devices, Heart & Vascular Institute (Miller Family), Cleveland Clinic, Cleveland, Ohio, USA

AUTHORS

ALI BAK AL-HADITHI, MB BChir, BA(Hons)
UCLA Cardiac Arrhythmia Center, David Geffen School of Medicine at UCLA, UCLA Health System, Los Angeles, California, USA

RYAN AZARRAFIY, BA
University of Miami Miller School of Medicine, Miami, Florida, USA

JAMIL BASHIR, MD, FRCS(C)
Clinical Associate Professor, University of British Columbia, St. Paul's Hospital, Vancouver, British Columbia, Canada

ULRIKA BIRGERSDOTTER-GREEN, MD
University of California, San Diego Medical Center, La Jolla, California, USA

NOEL G. BOYLE, MD, PhD, FHRS, FACC
Professor of Medicine, UCLA Cardiac Arrhythmia Center, David Geffen School of Medicine at UCLA, Ronald Reagan UCLA Medical Center, UCLA Health System, Los Angeles, California, USA

ROGER G. CARRILLO, MD, MBA, FHRS
Chief of Surgical Electrophysiology, The
Heart Institute at Palmetto General Hospital,
Hialeah, Florida, USA; Professor, University of
Miami Miller School of Medicine, Miami,
Florida, USA

DANIEL C. DeSIMONE, MD
Division of Infectious Diseases, Departments of
Medicine and Cardiovascular Diseases, Mayo
Clinic College of Medicine & Science,
Rochester, Minnesota, USA

DUC H. DO, MD
UCLA Cardiac Arrhythmia Center,
David Geffen School of Medicine at UCLA,
UCLA Health System, Los Angeles, California,
USA

MOHAMED B. ELSHAZLY, MD
Division of Cardiology, Department of
Medicine, Weill Cornell Medical College,
Doha, Qatar

MATTHEW FISCHER, MD
Assistant Clinical Professor, Department of
Anesthesiology and Perioperative Medicine,
David Geffen School of Medicine at UCLA,
Ronald Reagan UCLA Medical Center, UCLA
Health System, Los Angeles, California, USA

REED HARVEY, MD
Assistant Clinical Professor, Department of
Anesthesiology and Perioperative Medicine,
David Geffen School of Medicine at UCLA,
Ronald Reagan UCLA Medical Center, UCLA
Health System, Los Angeles, California, USA

JONATHAN K. HO, MD
Associate Clinical Professor, Department of
Anesthesiology and Perioperative Medicine,
David Geffen School of Medicine at UCLA,
Ronald Reagan UCLA Medical Center, UCLA
Health System, Los Angeles, California,
USA

KEVIN P. JACKSON, MD
Associate Professor of Medicine, Duke
University Medical Center, Durham, North
Carolina, USA

AKBAR H. KHAN, MD
United Heart & Vascular Clinic, Allina Health
System, St Paul, Minnesota, USA

FELIX KRAINSKI, MD
University of California, San Diego Medical
Center, La Jolla, California, USA

**CHARLES J. LOVE, MD, FACC, FAHA, FHRS,
CCDS**
Professor of Medicine, Director, Cardiac
Rhythm Device Services, The Johns Hopkins
Hospital, Baltimore, Maryland, USA

SANDEEP G. NAIR, MD
Cedars-Sinai Smidt Heart Institute, Los
Angeles, California, USA

VICTOR PRETORIUS, MBChB
University of California, San Diego Medical
Center, La Jolla, California, USA

MUHAMMAD RIZWAN SOHAIL, MD
Division of Infectious Diseases, Departments
of Medicine and Cardiovascular Diseases,
Mayo Clinic College of Medicine and Science,
Rochester, Minnesota, USA

CHARLES D. SWERDLOW, MD
Clinical Professor of Medicine, Cedars-Sinai
Smidt Heart Institute, Los Angeles, California,
USA

IMRAN S. SYED, MD
United Heart & Vascular Clinic, Allina
Health System, St Paul, Minnesota, USA

KHALDOUN G. TARAKJI, MD, MPH
Department of Cardiac Electrophysiology
and Pacing, Heart & Vascular Institute (Miller
Family), Cleveland Clinic, Cleveland, Ohio,
USA

PIERCE J. VATTEROTT, MD
United Heart & Vascular Clinic, Allina Health
System, St Paul, Minnesota, USA

**BRUCE L. WILKOFF, MD, FHRS, FACC,
FAHA, CCDS**
Professor of Medicine, Cleveland Clinic
Lerner College of Medicine of Case
Western Reserve University, Robert and
Suzanne Tomsich Department of
Cardiovascular Medicine, Director,
Cardiac Pacing and Tachyarrhythmia
Devices, Heart & Vascular Institute (Miller
Family), Cleveland Clinic, Cleveland, Ohio,
USA

Contents

> Lead management describes a comprehensive approach to cardiac implantable electronic device lead utilization, encompassing lead and device selection, vascular access, implant techniques, handling lead failures and recalls, managing infectious and other complications, and performing device and lead extraction. Device and lead selection should be based on the latest guidelines and the available data to choose the optimal device system for each patient. Lead extraction is a highly specialized procedure and should be carried out by a team of personnel extensively trained in the procedure at centers with cardiac surgical support.

Lead Management

> Transvenous approaches for pacemaker and defibrillator lead insertion offer numerous advantages over epicardial techniques. Although the cephalic, axillary, and subclavian veins are most commonly used in clinical practice, they each offer their own set of advantages and disadvantages that leave their usage dependent on patient anatomy and physician preference. Alternative methods using the upper and lower venous circulation have been described when these veins are not available or practical for lead insertion. Until current technology is superseded by leadless pacing systems, the search for the optimal lead insertion technique continues.

> The predominant structural mechanisms of transvenous lead dysfunction (LD) are conductor fracture and insulation breach. LD typically presents as an abnormality of electrical performance; the earliest sign usually is either oversensing or out-of-range pacing or shock impedance. Accurate diagnosis of LD requires discriminating patterns of oversensing and impedance trends that are characteristic of LD from similar patterns that occur in other conditions. Implantable cardioverter-defibrillators have advanced features to detect and mitigate the consequences of LD; these features operate both independently and in conjunction with remote monitoring networks.

Cardiovascular implantable electronic devices (CIEDs) and the indications for their use have significantly risen over the past decades to include patients who are older with more medical comorbidities. Predictably, the rates of CIED infection have increased substantially. CIED infection is associated with high morbidity, mortality, and financial costs. This article discusses the appropriate management of CIED infections, which is imperative to limit the problems associated with infection.

Lead Removal

Quality has a foundation that consists of the nomenclature, definitions, and metrics of success, failure, and complications. There is now a firm foundation for reporting outcomes and for making clinical decisions with patients and their families. This has developed from an international consensus, ratified by the four continental heart rhythm societies and by the overlapping cardiovascular, surgical, anesthesiology, and infectious disease societies. Reporting of outcomes, using these metrics and definitions, is now mandated to promote transparency and facilitate clinical decision making with patients. The best path to accomplishing this goal is to participate in a center-specific or multicenter registry.

The role of the anesthesiologist in lead extraction procedures is multifaceted and highlights the collaborative, multidisciplinary teamwork needed to ensure patient safety and procedural success in these complex cases. Thorough preoperative evaluation and identification of high-risk characteristics enable the anesthesiologist to tailor a comprehensive intraoperative and postoperative care plan for each case. Institutional practices may vary but anesthetic management typically includes general anesthesia with an endotracheal tube, invasive measurement of arterial blood pressure, vascular access for rapid volume expansion, echocardiographic monitoring, preparation for blood transfusion, and initiation of cardiopulmonary bypass in the event of an emergency.

Lead extraction procedures have a low but real risk of major complications, such as superior vena cava tear and cardiac tamponade. Complications during lead removal are commonly related to lead binding sites, lead malposition, and lead perforation. Lead extraction imaging may indicate lead vascular binding sites, lead position, and perforation. Several imaging modalities are available, including chest radiograph, cardiac computed tomography, and echocardiography. The information provided by various imaging modalities will help assess the challenges of each lead extraction procedure and allows for better preprocedure planning.

Removal of cardiovascular implantable electronic devices (CIED) is an important and growing field when managing patients presenting with device infections, need for upgrades, and lead failure. The complex skillset of transvenous lead removal is in high demand along with increasing numbers of implanted CIEDs. A systematic and comprehensive approach to this field, including knowledge of all available tools and vascular access techniques is essential for successful outcomes. This article serves as a practical resource presenting tools and techniques of transvenous lead extraction to help refine and master one's skill.

The rise in indications for cardiac implantable electronic devices has necessitated the development of tools for removal of the electrodes that connect the heart to these externally located pacemakers and defibrillators. After implant of a cardiac electrode, variable but progressive fibrous adhesion occurs. Removal of these adhesions can cause devastating complications with high risk of mortality if not treated surgically in a highly expeditious and appropriate manner. This article describes the incidence, risk factors, and diagnosis of these injuries followed by discussion of recent evidence for use of superior vena cava balloon occlusion, and conventional surgical repair of these injuries.

Surgical and hybrid lead extraction has developed considerably over the past several decades. Although transvenous lead extraction is the standard approach to remove infected or malfunctioning cardiac implantable electronic device leads, surgical approaches may be necessary in complex cases not amenable to transvenous lead extraction or in cases that involve concomitant pathologies, such as tricuspid valve regurgitation. We describe our experience with 4 minimally invasive surgical approaches to lead extraction as well as our experience with hybrid open heart surgery and transvenous lead extraction as an option for patients who present with concomitant conditions.

Patient Management

The number of implanted cardiovascular implantable electronic devices (CIEDs) has increased significantly in the last 30 years, which has led to an upsurge in CIED complications, such as infection and lead malfunction requiring CIED extraction. The decision-making process of CIED reimplantation requires meticulous planning that includes careful consideration of several aspects: the reason for extraction, the indication for CIED reimplantation, patients' wishes, timing of reimplantation, the need for a bridging device, and the type and location of device to be reimplanted. In this article, the authors review this decision-making process and the necessary steps to achieve optimal patient outcomes.

Video content accompanies this article at http://www.cardiacep.theclinics.com/.

With expanding indications for cardiac resynchronization therapy and increased survival of patients with cardiovascular disease, the need for lead addition or revision in the presence of an existing implantable electronic device is likely to increase. Partial or complete venous occlusion is frequently encountered and can be a significant barrier to successful procedural outcomes. Percutaneous options, including subclavian venoplasty, can reduce the need for significantly more invasive and morbid procedures and can readily be learned by the implanting physician. Additional invasive techniques, such as coronary sinus venoplasty and stenting, can be useful in cases of difficult left ventricular lead placement.

Although definitive therapy for infected cardiac implantable electronic device systems requires removal of all hardware in the infected areas with extraction of intravascular components as well, there are situations where extraction is not available or appropriate. Palliative procedures and chronic suppressive antibiotics may be used in these cases. There are also options that may in some cases result in long-term freedom from infection.

CARDIAC ELECTROPHYSIOLOGY CLINICS

THE CLINICS ARE AVAILABLE ONLINE!
Access your subscription at:
www.theclinics.com

Foreword
Lead Management

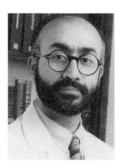   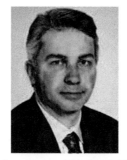

Ranjan K. Thakur, MD, MPH, MBA, FACC, FHRS   Andrea Natale, MD, FACC, FHRS
Consulting Editors

We are pleased to introduce this issue of *Cardiac Electrophysiology Clinics* on contemporary lead management issues in clinical practice.

Cardiac implantable electronic devices with leads have been implanted for over 60 years. These devices are getting ever more complex, and every few years a faulty lead with flaws and short lifespan is identified. Of course, device patients are living longer also; therefore, implanted leads are in their bodies longer, and there is more time for problems to develop.

We appreciate Drs Boyle and Wilkoff, who are leaders in this field, editing this issue of *Cardiac Electrophysiology Clinics*. They have divided this issue into general concepts and discussion about lead extraction. They have assembled a group of experts in the field, and together they have focused discussions on contemporary issues facing clinicians today.

We hope that the readers will enjoy reading these discussions, which may inform their own thinking and practice.

Ranjan K. Thakur, MD, MPH, MBA, FACC, FHRS
Sparrow Thoracic and Cardiovascular Institute
Michigan State University
1200 East Michigan Avenue, Suite 580
Lansing, MI 48912, USA

Andrea Natale, MD, FACC, FHRS
Texas Cardiac Arrhythmia Institute
Center for Atrial Fibrillation at
St. David's Medical Center
1015 East 32nd Street, Suite 516
Austin, TX 78705, USA

E-mail addresses:
thakur@msu.edu (R.K. Thakur)
andrea.natale@stdavids.com (A. Natale)

Card Electrophysiol Clin 10 (2018) xi
https://doi.org/10.1016/j.ccep.2018.09.002
1877-9182/18/© 2018 Published by Elsevier Inc.

Foreword

Lead Management

Rajan K. Thakur, MD, MPH, MBA, FACC, FHRS   Andrea Natale, MD, FACC, FHRS
Consulting Editors

Preface
Lead Management for Electrophysiologists

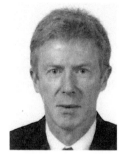
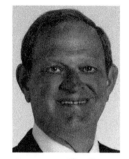

Noel G. Boyle, MD, PhD   Bruce L. Wilkoff, MD

Editors

The current issue of *Cardiac Electrophysiology Clinics* is focused on lead management, which encompasses all aspects of the care of patients with implanted pacemaker and ICD lead systems. It has been estimated that 1.2 million cardiac implantable electronic devices (CIEDs) are currently implanted annually worldwide. As the indications for CIED implant have expanded in recent decades, and the patient population gets older and has more comorbidities, complications associated with lead malfunction and device/lead-related infections continue to increase. The aim of this issue is to provide a review of lead management based on the most current best evidence, with the practical approach of leading experts working in the field.

Following an initial overview article, the first section of the issue focuses on lead management. Al-Hadithi and colleagues discuss vein management; Drs Nair and Swerdlow review electrode and lead design, and Sohail and associates discuss the approach to, and care of, device and lead infections. In the second section, attention is directed to lead removal techniques. Wilkoff and colleagues review definitions and metrics; Drs Birgersdotter-Green, Pretorius, and colleagues cover tools and techniques for lead extraction, while Bashir, Carrillo, and associates outline

extraction-related complications, recovery methods, and rescue surgery. Dr Fischer and associates review anesthetic considerations for lead extraction, and Vatterott and associates cover the role of imaging in lead management and patient care. The final section covers an array of topics in overall patient management. Tarakji and associates examine reimplantation after lead removal; Dr Jackson covers venoplasty and stenting, and Dr Love reviews palliation and nonextraction approaches. Carillo, Bashir, and colleagues discuss primary surgical and hybrid extraction methods.

While advances in device and lead design will continue in the coming decades, large numbers of patients with currently implanted leads and devices, and those undergoing device replacements and upgrades, will continue to need care and device and lead management during the course of their implants. We are confident that the state-of-the-art reviews provided in this issue, in addition to the recent Heart Rhythm Society and European Heart Rhythm Association guidelines, will provide a practical guide for improving clinical and procedure-related care and achieving optimal clinical outcomes for CIED patients.

The editors would like to thank the contributing authors for their comprehensive state-of-the-art

Card Electrophysiol Clin 10 (2018) xiii–xiv
https://doi.org/10.1016/j.ccep.2018.09.001
1877-9182/18/© 2018 Published by Elsevier Inc.

reviews, and the editorial staff at Elsevier for their excellent work in compiling and editing this issue.

Noel G. Boyle, MD, PhD
UCLA Cardiac Arrhythmia Center
Ronald Reagan UCLA Medical Center
David Geffen School of Medicine at UCLA
Los Angeles, CA 90095, USA

Bruce L. Wilkoff, MD
Director, Cardiac Pacing and Tachyarrhythmia
Devices
Robert and Suzanne Tomsich Department of
Cardiovascular Medicine
Sydell and Arnold Miller Family
Heart and Vascular Institute
Professor of Medicine
Cleveland Clinic Lerner College
of Medicine of CWRU
Cleveland Clinic
Cleveland, OH 44195, USA

E-mail addresses:
nboyle@mednet.ucla.edu (N.G. Boyle)
wilkofb@ccf.org (B.L. Wilkoff)

Overview of Lead Management

Noel G. Boyle, MD, PhD[a],*, Bruce L. Wilkoff, MD, CCDS[b]

KEYWORDS

- Vein management • Cardiac devices • Transvenous approaches • Laser lead extraction
- Mechanical lead extraction

KEY POINTS

- Lead management describes a comprehensive approach to cardiac implantable electronic device lead utilization, encompassing lead and device selection, vascular access, implant techniques, handling lead failures and recalls, managing infectious and other complications, and performing device and lead extraction.
- Device and lead selection should be based on the latest guidelines and the available data to choose the optimal device system for each patient.
- Lead extraction is a highly specialized procedure and should be carried out by a team of personnel extensively trained in the procedure at centers with cardiac surgical support.
- A full array of available tools, including mechanical and powered sheaths, locking stylets and snares, and ancillary equipment, should be available for every case.
- A team approach involving cardiac electrophysiologists, cardiac surgeons, cardiac anesthesiologists, with imaging and infectious disease specialists and technical staff is essential to ensuring optimal patient outcomes.

INTRODUCTION

In 2017, the Heart Rhythm Society (HRS) published an updated consensus statement on cardiac electronic implantable device (CIED) lead management and extraction (**Fig. 1, Tables 1–4**).[1] More recently, the European Heart Rhythm Association (EHRA) published the 2018 EHRA expert consensus on lead extraction, a similarly comprehensive overview of the field.[2] Both documents, authored by internationally recognized experts, provide a systematic, evidence-based, state-of-the-art overview of lead management and are referenced extensively in this review.

Lead extraction is defined as "any lead removal procedure in which at least one lead requires the assistance of equipment not typically required during implantation, or at least one lead was implanted for longer than one year."[1]

BACKGROUND

Since the first pacemaker implantation in 1958 and implantable cardioverter defibrillator (ICD) implantation in 1981, there has been rapid technological development in CIEDs with millions of these devices implanted worldwide. In the most recent world survey from 2009, an estimated 1,002,664 pacemakers were implanted, of which 737,840 were new implants and 264,824 were device replacements.[3] In the same year, there were 328,027 ICD implants, with 222,407 new implants and 105,620 replacements. Virtually all countries

[a] UCLA Cardiac Arrhythmia Center, UCLA Health System, David Geffen School of Medicine at UCLA, 100 UCLA Medical Plaza, Suite 660, Los Angeles, CA 90095, USA; [b] Robert and Suzanne Tomsich Department of Cardiovascular Medicine, Sydell and Arnold Miller Family Heart and Vascular Institute, Cleveland Clinic Lerner College of Medicine of CWRU, Cleveland Clinic, 9500 Euclid Avenue, Cleveland, OH 44195, USA
* Corresponding author.
E-mail address: nboyle@mednet.ucla.edu

Card Electrophysiol Clin 10 (2018) 549–559
https://doi.org/10.1016/j.ccep.2018.05.001

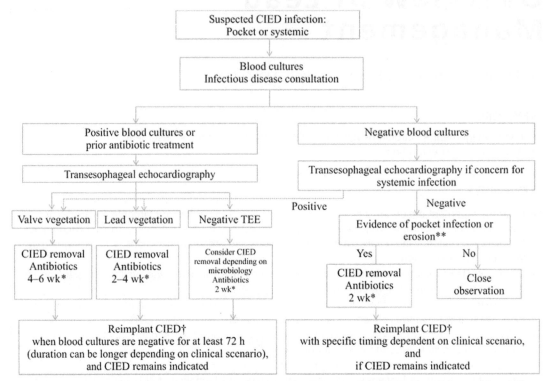

Fig. 1. Management of suspected CIED infection (flow chart). TEE, transesophageal echocardiography. * Refer to HRS expert consensus statement text for specific recommendations depending on microbiology. Antimicrobial therapy should be at least 4–6 weeks for endocarditis (4 weeks for native valve, 6 weeks for prosthetic valve or staphylococcal valvular endocarditis). If lead vegetation is present in the absence of a valve vegetation, 4 weeks of antibiotics for Staphylococcus aureus and 2 weeks for other pathogens is recommended. ** 2010 AHA CIED Infection Update distinguishes between pocket infection and erosion (Baddour et al. Circulation 2010;121:458–77). † Usually the contralateral side; a subcutaneous ICD may also be considered. (*From* Kusumoto FM, Schoenfeld MH, Wilkoff BL, et al. 2017 HRS expert consensus statement on cardiovascular implantable electronic device lead management and extraction. Heart Rhythm 2017;14:e521; with permission.)

showed a significant increase in device implants, particularly in ICDs, compared with a prior survey in 2005. The most recent estimates are that 1.2 to 1.4 million CIEDs are implanted annually worldwide.[1] In addition, from 1993 to 2009, implants of pacemakers in the United States increased yearly, with more dual-chamber devices being implanted in older patients with more comorbidities.[4] Over the last 2 decades, the implant indication for ICDs and cardiac resynchronization therapy (CRT) devices, with a pacemaker or with an ICD, have continued to expand, particularly with the proven benefits in patients with heart failure.[5–7] Furthermore, as patients with devices survive longer, more replacements and upgrades are being performed.[8]

Although both early pacers and ICDs were implanted surgically with epicardial leads, transvenous pacing leads became widely available in the 1960s for pacemakers and in the 1990s for ICDs and represent most implanted leads. Even as the devices themselves have become highly reliable, transvenous leads remain the Achilles heel of CIED systems. Lead failure rates range from 1% to 8% within 5 years of implantation, increasing with lead complexity such as in ICD leads. Notably higher failure rates have been reported for the Medtronic Sprint Fidelis lead (Medtronic, Minneapolis, MN) (2.6% per year) and the St. Jude Riata lead (St. Jude Medical [Abbott], Saint Paul, MN) (2.7% per year).[9] Fortunately, high transvenous lead extraction success rates for recalled leads have also been reported.[10,11]

LEAD MANAGEMENT

Lead management describes a comprehensive approach to CIED lead utilization, encompassing lead and device selection, implant techniques, vascular approaches, infectious complications, and device and lead extraction. The device, lead system, and implantation indication must

Table 1
Indications for lead extraction (noninfectious)

Class	Recommendations
Thrombosis/vascular issues	
I	Lead removal is recommended for patients with clinically significant thromboembolic events attributable to thrombus on a lead or a lead fragment that cannot be treated by other means.
I	Lead removal is recommended for patients with SVC stenosis or occlusion that prevents implantation of a necessary field.
I	Lead removal is recommended for patients with planned stent deployment in a vein already containing a transvenous lead, to avoid entrapment of the lead.
I	Lead removal as part of a comprehensive plan for maintaining patency is recommended for patients with SVC stenosis or occlusion with limiting symptoms.
IIa	Lead removal can be useful for patients with ipsilateral venous occlusion preventing access to the venous circulation for required placement of an additional lead.
Chronic pain	
IIa	Device and/or lead removal can be useful for patients with severe chronic pain at the device or lead insertion site or thought to be secondary to the device, which causes significant patient discomfort, is not manageable by medical or surgical techniques, and for which there is no acceptable alternative.
Other	
I	Lead removal is recommended for patients with life-threatening arrhythmias secondary to retained leads.
IIa	Lead removal can be useful for patients with a CIED location that interferes with the treatment of malignancy.
IIa	Lead removal can be useful for patients if a CIED implantation would require more than 4 leads on one side or more than 5 leads through the SVC.
IIa	Lead removal can be useful for patients with an abandoned lead that interferes with the operation of a CIED system.
IIb	Lead removal may be considered for patients with leads that, due to their design or their failure, pose a potential future threat to patients if left in place.
IIb	Lead removal may be considered for patients to facilitate access to MRI.
IIb	Lead removal may be considered in the setting of normally functioning nonrecalled pacing or defibrillation leads for selected patients after a shared decision-making process.

Abbreviation: SVC, superior vena cava.
Adapted from Kusumoto FM, Schoenfeld MH, Wilkoff BL, et al. 2017 HRS expert consensus statement on cardiovascular implantable electronic device lead management and extraction. Heart Rhythm 2017;14:e503–51; with permission.

be matched carefully with the indication, considering the most current guidelines, so that patients receive the optimal device system without exposing patients to unwarranted risks.[12–14] An example is the choice of a dual-versus single-coil ICD lead. When originally introduced in the late 1990s, dual-coil leads were reported to lower the defibrillation threshold compared with single-coil systems. This information was later questioned, with no clinically significant benefit found in a recent large national study.[15] However, it has been known for some time that leads with superior vena cava (SVC) coils are difficult and riskier to extract.[16] Hence, the risks and benefits of a dual-coil ICD lead should be carefully considered, particularly in younger patients. Similarly, active fixation leads, using a helical screw to secure the lead in position, are often easier to extract compared with the passive fixation tined leads, which often have more reactive tissue growth around the tines. Interestingly, it has never been proven that there is greater risk to removing passive fixation leads.

LEAD IMPLANTS

Lead implant techniques are correlated to device system infection and lead malfunction. Minimizing the risk of infection with preoperative removal of unnecessary indwelling central lines and catheters and assessment for current bacterial infections is

Table 2
Indications for lead extraction (infectious)

Class	Recommendations
I	If antibiotics are going to be prescribed, drawing at least 2 sets of blood cultures before starting antibiotic therapy is recommended for all patients with suspected CIED infection to improve the precision and minimize the duration of antibiotic therapy.
I	Gram stain and culture of generator pocket tissue and the explanted leads are recommended at the time of CIED removal to improve the precision and minimize the duration of antibiotic therapy.
I	Preprocedural TEE is recommended for patients with suspected systemic CIED infection to evaluate the absence or size, character, and potential embolic risk of identified vegetations.
I	Evaluation by physicians with specific expertise in CIED infection and lead extraction is recommended for patients with documented CIED infection.
IIa	TEE can be useful for patients with CIED pocket infection with and without positive blood cultures to evaluate the absence or size, character, and potential embolic risk of identified vegetations.
IIa	Evaluation by physicians with specific expertise in CIED infection and lead extraction can be useful for patients with suspected CIED infections.
IIb	Additional imaging may be considered to facilitate the diagnosis of CIED pocket or lead infection when it cannot be confirmed by other methods.

Abbreviation: TEE, transesophageal echocardiography.
Adapted from Kusumoto FM, Schoenfeld MH, Wilkoff BL, et al. 2017 HRS expert consensus statement on cardiovascular implantable electronic device lead management and extraction. Heart Rhythm 2017;14:e503–51; with permission.

crucial. A history of prior indwelling catheters may increase risk of vascular occlusion on the ipsilateral side, and a preprocedure venogram is valuable in establishing if the venous system on the preferred side is patent. The approach to patients with a dialysis fistula should first be discussed with the patients' nephrologist, and usually the contralateral side is used. Delaying prophylactic ICD placement until a mature fistula is in place may prevent infections stemming from chronic dialysis catheter use. Although most devices are implanted in cardiac catheterization or cardiac electrophysiology (EP) laboratories, meticulous attention to sterile techniques, similar to an operating room level, is required. The value of prophylactic antibiotics given within 1 hour of the start of the procedure is well established, with intravenous cephalosporin or vancomycin being the most commonly used prophylactic agents.[17,18] A large multicenter study of 1744 patients undergoing

Table 3
Risk factors for cardiovascular implantable electronic device infection

Patient-Related Factors	Procedure-Related Factors	Microbe-Related Factors
Age	Pocket reintervention (generator change, upgrade, lead or pocket revision)	Highly virulent microbes (eg, staphylococci)
Chronic kidney disease		
Hemodialysis		
Diabetes mellitus	Pocket hematoma	
Heart failure	Longer procedure duration	
Chronic obstructive pulmonary disease	Inexperienced operator	
	ICD (compared with PM)	
Preprocedure fever	Lack of use of prophylactic antibiotics	
Malignancy		
Skin disorder		
Immunosuppressive drug		
Prior CIED infection		
Anticoagulation		

Abbreviations: ICD, implantable cardioverter defibrillator; PM, pacemaker.
Adapted from Kusumoto FM, Schoenfeld MH, Wilkoff BL, et al. 2017 HRS expert consensus statement on cardiovascular implantable electronic device lead management and extraction. Heart Rhythm 2017;14:e503–51; with permission.

Table 4
Factors associated with extraction procedure complications and longer-term mortality

Factor	Associated Risk
Age	1.05-fold ↑ mortality
Female sex	4.5-fold ↑ risk of major complications
Low body mass index (<25 kg/m²)	1.8-fold ↑ risk of 30-d mortality ↑ number of procedure-related complications
History of cerebrovascular accident	2-fold ↑ risk of major complications
Severe LV dysfunction	2-fold ↑ risk of major complications
Advanced HF	1.3- to 8.5-fold ↑ risk of 30-d mortality 3-fold ↑ 1-y mortality
Renal dysfunction	ESRD: 4.8-fold ↑ risk of 30-d mortality Cr ≥2.0: ↑ in-hospital mortality and 2-fold ↑ risk 1-y mortality
Diabetes mellitus	↑ in-hospital mortality 1.71-fold ↑ mortality
Platelet count	Low platelet count: 1.7 fold ↑ risk of major complications
Coagulopathy	Elevated INR: 2.7-fold ↑ risk of major complications and 1.3 fold ↑ risk of 30-d mortality
Anemia	3.3-fold ↑ risk of 30-d mortality
Number of leads extracted	3.5-fold ↑ risk of any complication 1.6-fold ↑ long-term mortality
Presence of dual-coil ICD	2.7-fold ↑ risk of 30-d mortality
Extraction for infection	2.7- to 30.0-fold ↑ risk of 30-d mortality 5.0- to 9.7-fold ↑ 1-y mortality CRP >72 mg/L associated with ↑ 30-d mortality 3.52-fold ↑ mortality
Operator experience	2.6-fold ↑ number of procedure-related complications
Prior open heart surgery	↓ risk of major complications

Abbreviations: Cr, creatinine; CRP, C-reactive protein; ESRD, end-stage renal disease; HF, heart failure; ICD, implantable cardioverter defibrillator; INR, international normalized ratio; LV, left ventricular.

Adapted from Kusumoto FM, Schoenfeld MH, Wilkoff BL, et al. 2017 HRS expert consensus statement on cardiovascular implantable electronic device lead management and extraction. Heart Rhythm 2017;14:e503–51; with permission.

device replacements at 72 US sites found a low infection rate of 1.3%.[19]

Venous access may be obtained using the cephalic vein (cut-down) or the axillary or subclavian veins (Seldinger technique). The cephalic approach avoids the risk of pneumothorax, but small vein size may limit the number of leads. The axillary approach has the advantage of being an extrathoracic puncture, whereas the more medial subclavian approach has a higher incidence of pneumothorax and lead crush between the first rib and the clavicle.[20] When the leads are fixed in place, it is important to leave adequate, but not excessive, slack to compensate deep breathing in the standing position. The leads should be firmly sutured in placed using the suture sleeves, taking care not to damage the insulation with excessively tight sutures. For younger patients, a subcutaneous pocket will usually provide adequate tissue support for the device can, but with the risk of increased mechanical lead failures, whereas a submuscular pocket may provide a preferred cosmetic result, particularly with ICD devices. However, in more elderly and thinner patients with little subcutaneous tissue, an intramuscular or submuscular device pocket will decrease the risk of later device erosion and in addition provide a better cosmetic result for patients.

Attention to hemostasis is essential in closing the pocket, as bleeding and hematomas increase risk of infection and reoperation. It is now well established that device implantation without interruption of warfarin anticoagulation significantly reduced device pocket hematoma when compared with a heparin bridging strategy.[21,22] Currently, novel oral anticoagulants are typically held for 24 hours before device implantation; this approach has not been associated with an increased risk of bleeding or thromboembolic events.[23] Compression dressings should be considered in patients on anticoagulation following device implants or revisions.

LEAD FAILURES

Lead failures/malfunctions are responsible for 20% of device extractions in a large single-center study in 2009 and 38% in the EHRA large multicenter study (the European Lead Extraction Controlled Registry [ELECTRa]) reported in 2017.[24,25] The most prominent lead failures in the last decade have been the Fidelis Lead (Medtronic Inc, Minneapolis, MN), recalled in October 2007, and the Riata Lead, recalled in November 2011. Although both leads were the focus of FDA class I recall, mandating that no further implants of the leads could be performed, this did not necessarily require that the leads needed to be removed or replaced. Typically, the initial clinical approach involves more intensive monitoring of the leads including remote monitoring, with decisions to continue monitoring, replace and or extract and replace the lead taken after detailed discussions with the patient on the risks and benefits of each approach with the patient. The HRS' current 2017 guidelines emphasize the importance on shared decision-making with the patients considering the consequences of lead failure and the operative risks.[1]

More than 90% of the Fidelis lead failures were caused by a fracture of one or more pace-sense conductors, most commonly in the cable to the ring electrode distally.[26] In this comprehensive review on lead failures, Swerdlow and colleagues[26] state that the root cause was related to the extreme flexibility of the Fidelis lead, which allowed bending with a short radius of curvature, resulting in high stress to the metal components. In contrast, for the Riata leads with silicone-only insulation, abrasions resulting in external (outside-in) or internal (inside-out) insulation breaches were the primary cause of lead failures. Most commonly, these inside-out abrasions presented as externalized cables between the shock coils that could be identified radiologically.[27] However, externalization of the conductors usually does not result in electrical failure and depending on the age of patients and comorbid conditions, continued use of a Riata is often possible.

DEVICE AND LEAD INFECTIONS

Infections of the CIED system with device pocket, lead, or endocarditis accounted for approximately 60% of lead extractions in the 2009 study from Kennergren and colleagues[24] and 53% in the EHRA ELECTRa registry in 2017.[24,25] Of these, an estimated 60% are related to local/pocket infections and 40% due to systemic infection (sepsis and endocarditis).[24,28] In the large observational study from the Cleveland clinic, Tarakji and coworkers[28] reported on 412 consecutive patients in a 5-year period from 2002 to 2007. In this cohort, 220 (53%) patients had a permanent pacemaker, 126 (31%) had an ICD, and 66 (16%) had a CRT device. The average number of leads was 2.4 per patient, and the median time from device implant or replacement was 469 days. Of 414 pathogens isolated, 88% were aerobic gram positive, 9% were aerobic gram-negative organisms, with the remainder comprising anaerobes, fungi, and mycobacterium species. Ninety percent of the aerobic gram-positive organisms were staphylococci, of which 45% were *Staphylococcus aureus* and 55% coagulase-negative staphylococci. Approximately half of both staphylococcal species were methicillin resistant. Similar findings were reported by Sohail and coworkers[29] in a retrospective study of 189 patients with device infections seen at the Mayo Clinic from 1991 to 2003 (**Fig. 2**).

In the case of evident pocket infections with pus drainage, erosions, or extrusions, the diagnosis is readily apparent. (**Fig. 3**) However, the diagnosis is

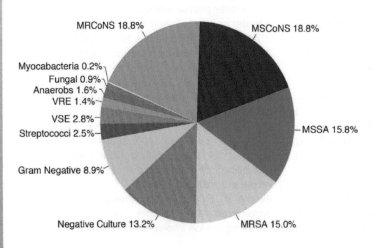

Fig. 2. Microbiology of CIED infections. *S aureus, Staphylococcus aureus.* (*From* Sohail MR, Uslan DZ, Khan AH, et al. Management and outcome of permanent pacemaker and implantable cardioverter-defibrillator infections. Journal of the American College of Cardiology 2007; 49(18):1853; with permission.)

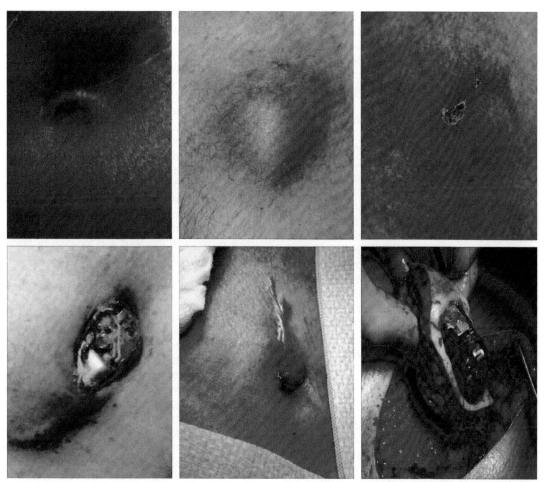

Fig. 3. Examples of device-related pocket infections displaying a range of abnormal appearances. (*From* Padfield GJ, Steinberg C, Bennett MT, et al. Preventing cardiac implantable electronic device infections. Heart Rhythm 2015;12:2347; with permission.)

often delayed in patients presenting with fever, chills, and an intact pocket, whereby positive blood cultures and/or echocardiographic evidence of vegetations are required to make the diagnosis. Approximately one-fifth of patients presenting with an apparent pocket infection also had evidence of bacteremia, and up to half of those who underwent a transesophageal echocardiogram had evidence of vegetations. Patients with systemic infection were more likely to have systemic comorbidities, such as diabetes or renal failure. The investigators emphasized that pocket infections and endovascular infections should be considered a continuum and that device removal is needed to eradicate the infection.

CIED infections are associated with a high morbidity and mortality. Although the extraction-related mortality was low (0.5%) in this highly experienced center, the in-hospital mortality was 4.6%. Overall, the 1-year mortality was 12% for the pocket-infection group and 25% for the endovascular-infection group (overall 17%). Reimplantation was deferred, when possible, until the antibiotic treatment was completed; about one-third of patients did not require reimplantation during the hospitalization. In pacer-dependent patients, placement of a percutaneous active fixation lead via the jugular vein, connected to an external device battery, provides an effective option for bridging these patients until they are infection free and can receive a new permanent implant.[30] This approach has the added advantage of allowing patient mobility and not requiring intensive care unit (ICU) monitoring.

Several recent studies have found that as the rate and complexity of CIED implants has increased with expanding indications, so also has the rate of device-related infections.[31] This finding also reflects an older and sicker patient population undergoing more frequent and higher-risk procedures.[32] Multiple comorbidities, such as immunosuppression, chronic steroid use, anticoagulant and/or antiplatelet therapy, diabetes, heart failure, renal insufficiency, chronic obstructive pulmonary disease, chronic malignancy and advanced age often present in this patient population, further increase infection risk. Procedure-related factors associated with increased risk include additional leads, hematoma, device revision, and operator experience. Although ongoing studies are evaluating the role of novel approaches, such as intensified antibiotic therapy or a bioresorbable antibacterial mesh in the pocket, attention to detail in managing comorbid conditions and implant surgery offers the best opportunities to reduce device-related infections. It is important to note that although it is possible to predict increased risk of infection and it is possible to predict poor long-term outcomes after treatment of CIED infection,[33] both related to comorbid conditions, the risk of transvenous lead extraction is low even in patients with old and multiple leads. The risk of extraction is extremely low, especially in comparison with outcomes related to CIED infection.

FACILITY REQUIREMENTS

Lead extraction has low-frequency but potentially life-threatening complications. A strong institutional commitment and vigilance is require to develop and maintain a team with expertise and training.[1,2] Similar outcomes have been shown whether the procedure is performed in a cardiac catheterization laboratory or operating room; the key requirement is that the location has all necessary equipment to perform the extraction safely and deal with any complications.[34] Given that a complication, such as SVC tear or cardiac perforation, may be catastrophic, it is critical that a cardiac surgeon and full support team including perfusionist and equipment be available to provide emergency open chest surgical repair within 5 to 10 minutes.[35] The recent availability of a compliant SVC occlusion balloon to manage SVC tears provides only short hemostasis and hemodynamic support.[36] Appropriate individual and team training for all staff is the key to maximal procedure success and minimal procedural complications and to successful outcomes when serious complications arise. Current guidelines from the HRS and EHRA recommend 30 lead extractions as the minimal volume to achieve clinical competence.[37] Simulation training may also provide valuable additional experience when the procedure volume is not high.[38]

PREPROCEDURE, INTRAPROCEDURE, AND POSTPROCEDURE CONSIDERATIONS
Preprocedure

A complete patient history and examination with laboratory and cardiac evaluations are required to prepare for a safe and effective extraction procedure. The indication for extraction, initial indication for CIED, pacemaker dependence, and any antibiotic therapy received should be established. The type of device and all leads present, date of implant, fixation mechanism, and lead location should be ascertained. Blood tests should include hemoglobin, platelet count, coagulation tests, renal function, and blood cultures if an infection is suspected. Imaging studies should include a chest radiograph (number and location of leads, calcification), echocardiography (ejection fraction, valve function, vegetations, intracardiac shunt, any pericardial fluid), and contrast venography/computed tomography (vein stenosis/occlusion, extravascular lead segments) if indicated.[2] A transesophageal echocardiography (TEE) may also be indicated to further clarify the vegetation size; current data support a percutaneous extraction approach for vegetations up to 4 cm in size (usually <2.5 cm) and consideration of a surgical approach for larger than this.[39,40] Female patients, a body mass index less than 25 kg/m^2, higher number of leads, leads greater than 10 years old, and dual-coil leads are all indications for more difficult procedures.[35,41] In addition, this information can be used to construct a lead extraction difficulty index to predict potential complexity of the procedure.[42] Although it is not possible to predict who is going to have a procedural complication, it is possible to determine the 30-day survival rate by 10 clinical parameters developed into a nomogram.[33] The net procedural major complication rate and the net procedural mortality rate have consistently been, even in complex procedures, less than 2%.

Intraprocedure

The location (operating room, hybrid room, or catheterization laboratory) and type of anesthesia should be clarified. The intraoperative imaging needed (fluoroscopy, TEE) should be present in the room. The personnel present should include cardiac EP, cardiac surgeon, cardiac anesthesiologist (with TEE experience), perfusion staff, radiological technician, and operating room and catheterization laboratory staff familiar with lead extraction equipment (mechanical and laser sheaths; consider snares, bridge balloon). A time-out review of the case with the anticipated risk of complications and response plan should be fully discussed, with roles and responsibilities clearly defined. If temporary backup pacing is needed, the authors prefer to use a temporary pacing wire from the femoral vessel during the procedure and a permanent transvenous lead connected to an external device for increased stability postoperatively.[30] For cases deemed very high risk, the authors also prefer to have 4 units of blood in the extraction procedure room. If reimplantation is needed, all equipment and support staff should be available. The success of extraction for each lead is defined as complete, partial (<4 cm remains in situ), or failure (>4 cm remains in situ).[1]

Postprocedure

Patients should be monitored at a level appropriate to overall/cardiac status (ICU, telemetry monitoring), with treatment of any intraoperative and postoperative complications and postextraction wound care. In patients with infected CIEDs who are pacemaker dependent, temporary backup pacing, as described earlier, may need to be continued until antibiotic therapy is completed and reimplantation can be undertaken. Discharge and follow-up planning should be initiated.

SUMMARY

Although technological advances, such as the subcutaneous ICD, may replace transvenous leads, new problems in device management may arise, such as how to remove a leadless pacemaker. However, for the foreseeable future, most implanted devices will still use transvenous leads and pectoral devices. The EHRA document has listed several gaps in evidence at present, such as effectiveness of different antibiotic strategies, developing better risk stratification, and what size of vegetation requires an open surgical approach.[2] Further evidence deficits include the lack of randomized trials, and limited registry data remain to be addressed.

The following articles in this text cover all aspects of lead management: venous access, lead characteristics, treatment of infections, extraction techniques, management of complications, surgical and hybrid approaches, the role of imaging and anesthesia, and palliation approaches.

REFERENCES

1. Kusumoto FM, Schoenfeld MH, Wilkoff BL, et al. 2017 HRS expert consensus statement on cardiovascular implantable electronic device lead management and extraction. Heart Rhythm 2017;14: e503–51.

2. Bongiorni MG, Burri H, Deharo JC, et al, ESC Scientific Document Group. 2018 EHRA expert consensus statement on lead extraction: recommendations on definitions, endpoints, research trial design, and data collection requirements for clinical scientific studies and registries: endorsed by APHRS/HRS/LAHRS. Europace 2018. [Epub ahead of print].

3. Mond HG, Proclemer A. The 11th world survey of cardiac pacing and implantable cardioverter-defibrillators: calendar year 2009–a World Society of Arrhythmia's project. Pacing Clin Electrophysiol 2011;34:1013–27.

4. Greenspon AJ, Patel JD, Lau E, et al. Trends in permanent pacemaker implantation in the United States from 1993 to 2009: increasing complexity of patients and procedures. J Am Coll Cardiol 2012;60:1540–5.

5. Goldberger Z, Lampert R. Implantable cardioverter-defibrillators: expanding indications and technologies. JAMA 2006;295:809–18.

6. Stevenson WG, Hernandez AF, Carson PE, et al, Heart Failure Society of America Guideline Committee. Indications for cardiac resynchronization therapy: 2011 update from the Heart Failure Society of America Guideline Committee. J Card Fail 2012; 18:94–106.

7. Normand C, Linde C, Singh J, et al. Indications for cardiac resynchronization therapy: a comparison of the major international guidelines. JACC Heart Fail 2018;6:308–16.

8. Essebag V, Joza J, Birnie DH, et al. Incidence, predictors, and procedural results of upgrade to resynchronization therapy: the RAFT upgrade substudy. Circ Arrhythm Electrophysiol 2015;8:152–8.

9. Fazal IA, Shepherd EJ, Tynan M, et al. Comparison of sprint fidelis and riata defibrillator lead failure rates. Int J Cardiol 2013;168:848–52.

10. El-Chami MF, Merchant FM, Levy M, et al. Outcomes of sprint fidelis and riata lead extraction: data from 2 high-volume centers. Heart Rhythm 2015;12:1216–20.

11. Brunner MP, Cronin EM, Jacob J, et al. Transvenous extraction of implantable cardioverter-defibrillator leads under advisory–a comparison of Riata, Sprint Fidelis, and non-recalled implantable cardioverter-defibrillator leads. Heart Rhythm 2013;10:1444–50.

12. Epstein AE, DiMarco JP, Ellenbogen KA, et al, American College of Cardiology/American Heart Association Task Force on Practice Guidelines (Writing Committee to Revise the ACC/AHA/NASPE 2002 Guideline Update for Implantation of Cardiac Pacemakers and Antiarrhythmia Devices), American Association for Thoracic Surgery; Society of Thoracic Surgeons. ACC/AHA/HRS 2008 guidelines for device-based therapy of cardiac rhythm abnormalities: a report of the American College of Cardiology/American Heart Association Task Force on Practice Guidelines (Writing Committee to Revise

the ACC/AHA/NASPE 2002 Guideline Update for Implantation of Cardiac Pacemakers and Antiarrhythmia Devices) developed in collaboration with the American Association for Thoracic Surgery and Society of Thoracic Surgeons. J Am Coll Cardiol 2008;51:e1–62.

13. Brignole M, Auricchio A, Baron-Esquivias G, et al. 2013 ESC Guidelines on cardiac pacing and cardiac resynchronization therapy: the Task Force on cardiac pacing and resynchronization therapy of the European Society of Cardiology (ESC). Developed in collaboration with the European Heart Rhythm Association (EHRA). Eur Heart J 2013;34: 2281–329.

14. Epstein AE, DiMarco JP, Ellenbogen KA, et al, American College of Cardiology Foundation, American Heart Association Task Force on Practice Guidelines, Heart Rhythm Society. 2012 ACCF/AHA/HRS focused update incorporated into the ACCF/AHA/HRS 2008 guidelines for device-based therapy of cardiac rhythm abnormalities: a report of the American College of Cardiology Foundation/American Heart Association Task Force on Practice Guidelines and the Heart Rhythm Society. J Am Coll Cardiol 2013;61:e6–75.

15. Larsen JM, Hjortshoj SP, Nielsen JC, et al. Single-coil and dual-coil defibrillator leads and association with clinical outcomes in a complete Danish nationwide ICD cohort. Heart Rhythm 2016;13:706–12.

16. Epstein LM, Love CJ, Wilkoff BL, et al. Superior vena cava defibrillator coils make transvenous lead extraction more challenging and riskier. J Am Coll Cardiol 2013;61:987–9.

17. Da Costa A, Kirkorian G, Cucherat M, et al. Antibiotic prophylaxis for permanent pacemaker implantation: a meta-analysis. Circulation 1998;97:1796–801.

18. Klug D, Balde M, Pavin D, et al, PEOPLE Study Group. Risk factors related to infections of implanted pacemakers and cardioverter-defibrillators: results of a large prospective study. Circulation 2007;116: 1349–55.

19. Uslan DZ, Gleva MJ, Warren DK, et al. Cardiovascular implantable electronic device replacement infections and prevention: results from the REPLACE registry. Pacing Clin Electrophysiol 2012;35:81–7.

20. Parsonnet V, Roelke M. The cephalic vein cutdown versus subclavian puncture for pacemaker/ICD lead implantation. Pacing Clin Electrophysiol 1999; 22:695–7.

21. Birnie DH, Healey JS, Wells GA, et al, BRUISE CONTROL Investigators. Pacemaker or defibrillator surgery without interruption of anticoagulation. N Engl J Med 2013;368:2084–93.

22. Pecha S, Ayikli A, Wilke I, et al. Bleeding risk of submuscular ICD implantation with continued oral anticoagulation versus heparin bridging therapy. Heart Vessels 2018;33:441–6.

23. Davies RA, Perera NK, Orr Y. Do novel anticoagulant agents increase the risk of perioperative complications during implantable cardiac rhythm device insertion? Interact Cardiovasc Thorac Surg 2017; 24:126–8.

24. Kennergren C, Bjurman C, Wiklund R, et al. A single-centre experience of over one thousand lead extractions. Europace 2009;11:612–7.

25. Bongiorni MG, Kennergren C, Butter C, et al, ELECTRa Investigators. The European Lead Extraction ConTRolled (ELECTRa) study: a European Heart Rhythm Association (EHRA) registry of transvenous lead extraction outcomes. Eur Heart J 2017;38: 2995–3005.

26. Swerdlow CD, Kalahasty G, Ellenbogen KA. Implantable cardiac defibrillator lead failure and management. J Am Coll Cardiol 2016;67:1358–68.

27. Hauser RG, McGriff D, Retel LK. Riata implantable cardioverter-defibrillator lead failure: analysis of explanted leads with a unique insulation defect. Heart Rhythm 2012;9:742–9.

28. Tarakji KG, Chan EJ, Cantillon DJ, et al. Cardiac implantable electronic device infections: presentation, management, and patient outcomes. Heart Rhythm 2010;7:1043–7.

29. Sohail MR, Uslan DZ, Khan AH, et al. Management and outcome of permanent pacemaker and implantable cardioverter-defibrillator infections. J Am Coll Cardiol 2007;49:1851–9.

30. Braun MU, Rauwolf T, Bock M, et al. Percutaneous lead implantation connected to an external device in stimulation-dependent patients with systemic infection–a prospective and controlled study. Pacing Clin Electrophysiol 2006;29:875–9.

31. Sohail MR, Henrikson CA, Braid-Forbes MJ, et al. Mortality and cost associated with cardiovascular implantable electronic device infections. Arch Intern Med 2011;171:1821–8.

32. Padfield GJ, Steinberg C, Bennett MT, et al. Preventing cardiac implantable electronic device infections. Heart Rhythm 2015;12:2344–56.

33. Brunner MP, Yu C, Hussein AA, et al. Nomogram for predicting 30-day all-cause mortality after transvenous pacemaker and defibrillator lead extraction. Heart Rhythm 2015;12:2381–6.

34. Franceschi F, Dubuc M, Deharo JC, et al. Extraction of transvenous leads in the operating room versus electrophysiology laboratory: a comparative study. Heart Rhythm 2011;8:1001–5.

35. Bernardes de Souza B, Benharash P, Esmailian F, et al. Value of a joint cardiac surgery-cardiac electrophysiology approach to lead extraction. J Card Surg 2015;30:874–6.

36. Wilkoff BL, Kennergren C, Love CJ, et al. Bridge to surgery: best practice protocol derived from early clinical experience with the bridge occlusion balloon. Federated Agreement from the Eleventh

Annual Lead Management Symposium. Heart Rhythm 2017;14:1574–8.

37. Zipes DP, Calkins H, Daubert JP, et al. 2015 ACC/AHA/HRS advanced training statement on clinical cardiac electrophysiology (a revision of the ACC/AHA 2006 update of the clinical competence statement on invasive electrophysiology studies, catheter ablation, and cardioversion). Heart Rhythm 2016;13:e3–37.

38. Maytin M, Daily TP, Carillo RG. Virtual reality lead extraction as a method for training new physicians: a pilot study. Pacing Clin Electrophysiol 2015;38:319–25.

39. Grammes JA, Schulze CM, Al-Bataineh M, et al. Percutaneous pacemaker and implantable cardioverter-defibrillator lead extraction in 100 patients with intracardiac vegetations defined by transesophageal echocardiogram. J Am Coll Cardiol 2010;55:886–94.

40. Maloney JD, Maloney JD 3rd. Vegetation size marker for extraction technique? J Am Coll Cardiol 2010;55:895–7.

41. Fermin L, Gebhard RE, Azarrafiy R, et al. Pearls of wisdom for high-risk laser lead extractions: a focused review. Anesth Analg 2018;126:406–12.

42. Bontempi L, Vassanelli F, Cerini M, et al. Predicting the difficulty of a transvenous lead extraction procedure: validation of the LED index. J Cardiovasc Electrophysiol 2017;28:811–8.

Lead Management

Vein Management for Cardiac Device Implantation

Ali BAK Al-Hadithi, MB BChir, Duc H. Do, MD,
Noel G. Boyle, MD, PhD*

KEYWORDS

- Vein management • Cardiac devices • Transvenous approaches • Lead insertion

KEY POINTS

- Cephalic cutdown and subclavian and axillary venipuncture are the most common techniques in clinical practice for transvenous pacemaker or defibrillator lead insertion.
- Venipuncture techniques can be facilitated by anatomic knowledge in conjunction with the use of fluoroscopy, contrast venography, and/or ultrasound.
- Alternative transvenous approaches have been described in cases in which cephalic, subclavian, and axillary veins are not available or practical for lead insertion. These include the external jugular, internal jugular, iliofemoral, supraclavicular subclavian, brachiocephalic, and azygos veins.
- Lead implantation via a persistent left superior vena cava, the most common venous anomaly of the thorax, can be technically difficult or impossible. Nevertheless, there have been numerous reports describing successful lead insertion using the subclavian vein and, more recently, a communicating branch between the anatomic anomaly and the right superior vena cava.

INTRODUCTION

Most pacemaker and implantable cardioverter-defibrillator (ICD) device leads are positioned endocardially through a transvenous approach. In comparison with epicardial approaches, transvenous lead placement offers several advantages: no requirement for general anesthesia, the option to use bipolar leads, lower complication rates, and lower costs.[1] The selection of veins for this procedure is influenced by patient anatomy, lead size, type of device, and physician preference. Due to relative ease of access and low complication rates, the cephalic, subclavian, and axillary veins are most commonly used in clinical practice. Indeed, the cephalic vein is the preferred first approach in 60% of European centers, whereas 40% use the subclavian or axillary vein.[2] In cases in which these veins are occluded or unusable,

the iliofemoral, internal jugular, external jugular, brachiocephalic, and azygos veins are alternative routes for lead placement.

VENOUS ANATOMY

The axillary vein is formed by the union of the brachial and basilic veins at the inferior border of the teres major muscle (**Fig. 1**). It receives the brachial vein near the lower border of subscapularis and passes under the pectoralis minor muscles to terminate at the outer border of the first rib, where it becomes the subclavian vein.

The cephalic vein is a superficial vein that runs on the anterolateral aspect of the forearm and arm. It passes between the deltoid and pectoralis major muscles (deltopectoral groove) near the shoulder. At the upper end of the deltopectoral groove, it pierces the clavicopectoral fascia to

UCLA Cardiac Arrhythmia Center, UCLA Health System, David Geffen School of Medicine at UCLA, 100 UCLA Medical Plaza, Los Angeles, CA 90095, USA
* Corresponding author.
E-mail address: nboyle@mednet.ucla.edu

Card Electrophysiol Clin 10 (2018) 561–571
https://doi.org/10.1016/j.ccep.2018.05.003
1877-9182/18/© 2018 Elsevier Inc. All rights reserved.

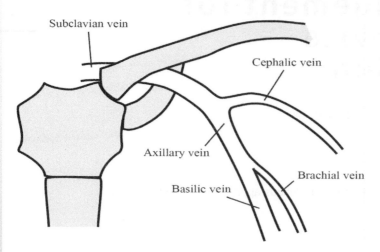

Subclavian vein

Cephalic vein

Axillary vein

Brachial vein

Basilic vein

Fig. 1. Line diagram showing anatomy of venous drainage in the left upper arm/shoulder area.

join the axillary vein just below the clavicle, together forming the subclavian vein.

The subclavian vein extends from the superior border of the first rib under and behind the clavicle. It runs alongside and anterior to the subclavian artery, which are separated from each other by the anterior scalene muscle. The brachial plexus lies superior to the subclavian artery. The external jugular vein joins the subclavian vein lateral or anterior to the anterior scalene muscle. At the medial border of the anterior scalene muscle, the internal jugular vein joins the subclavian vein to form the brachiocephalic vein. Both left and right brachiocephalic veins combine to drain into the heart as the superior vena cava.

The azygos vein is a unilateral, right-sided vessel that enters the thorax through the aortic hiatus (12th thoracic vertebral level) in the diaphragm. It ascends in the posterior mediastinum along the right side of the vertebral column until it reaches the right main bronchus, where it arches anteriorly to join into the superior vena cava.

Body habitus, shoulder movements, and skeletal deformities are factors that can greatly influence the anatomic relationship between the first rib and the clavicle.[3] In contrast, the relationship between the first rib and subclavian vein is constant.[4] It is important to note that high compression pressures may be exerted on leads lying between the first rib and clavicle, especially if they are entrapped by the costoclavicular ligaments.[5–9]

VENOUS APPROACHES: CUTDOWN AND VENIPUNCTURE

Venous access for lead implantation can be obtained through either cutdown or venipuncture methods. The depth and size of veins are the major factors that determine which technique should be used (**Table 1**).

Cutdown methods are most frequently used when the vein is superficial and of at least a moderate diameter. Exposing it by dissection will allow direct visualization, where it can be incised to permit lead entry.

Venipuncture methods can access deeper veins despite the lack of direct visualization. It is reserved for larger, deeper veins that are more amenable to needle entry, including the subclavian, axillary, and internal jugular veins. This avoids the issues surrounding dissection of such deep structures and, given their large diameter, are more likely to accommodate multiple leads. However, the lack of visualization increases the risk of damage to adjacent structures, be it vessels, nerves, or the pleural cavity. In addition, there is a possibility of inadvertent cannulation of a vessel adjacent to the intended target.[3]

Venous drainage is not significantly affected by venous cutdown and ligation of smaller veins (cephalic and external jugular), so they can be sacrificed during the procedure. In contrast, deeper veins (axillary and subclavian) serve sufficiently large territories such that venous drainage would be impaired by ligation; bleeding from these large veins is stemmed by pressure exerted from neighboring structures.[3]

CEPHALIC VEIN

The cephalic vein is amenable to cutdown techniques due to its superficial position in the deltopectoral groove. Once isolated from its surrounding tissue, the vein is ligated distally, and a ligature looped around the proximal segment. An incision is subsequently made between the proximal and distal ligatures to permit lead entry.

Cephalic vein access has little risk of damaging adjacent structures. By using the cutdown technique, the vein can be directly visualized for lead

Table 1
Summary of the advantages and disadvantages of the most commonly used veins for lead insertion

	Cephalic Vein	Subclavian Vein	Axillary Vein
Advantages	Little risk of damaging vital adjacent structures Does not require venography	Large size, so easier to insert leads and can accommodate multiple leads Accessible via venipuncture Anatomically close to the pulse generator site Quicker to perform	Large size, so easier to insert leads and can accommodate multiple leads Accessible via venipuncture Anatomically close to the pulse generator site Quicker to perform
Disadvantages	Time-consuming Success highly dependent on venous diameter, patency, and tortuosity Accommodates a maximum of 2 leads Lower rates of success	Cannot visualize directly Close to many vital structures, including the subclavian artery, brachial plexus, and phrenic nerve Risk of pneumothorax and hemo-pneumothorax Lead crush	Cannot visualize directly Close to many vital structures, including the subclavian artery, brachial plexus, and phrenic nerve

insertion and, as there are no adjacent vessels, the risk of entry into an incorrect vessel is minimal. In addition, although contrast venography is often used in clinical practice, it is not required for the success of this method.

Kolettis and colleagues[10] investigated refinements of the cutdown method: cannulation of retro-pectoral veins in cases of insufficient caliber, use of a hydrophilic guidewire when direct lead insertion failed, simultaneous use of 2 guidewires, and use of stiff angiography guidewires. They compared 200 patients undergoing the standard method with an equal cohort undergoing the refined methods. Results showed that the refinements group had a higher success rate at cephalic vein access (96% vs 80%). Fluoroscopy time, lead placement time, and complication rates were comparable between the 2 groups; although the refinements group had no major complications whereas the standard approach produced 5 cases (2.5%), the differences were not statistically significant.

However, the success rate of cephalic vein access is not as high as venipuncture.[11] Successful lead insertion in the cephalic vein may be observed in 64% to 96% of patients.[10–14] Several causes account for such a high rate of failure, the most common being the size and course of the cephalic vein, the presence of venous stenosis, or extensive vessel tortuosity.[14] Furthermore, accessing the cephalic vein can be time-consuming and it accommodates a maximum of 2 leads, so additional venous access is needed for biventricular pacing.

AXILLARY AND SUBCLAVIAN VEINS

The current conventional approach to axillary or subclavian venipuncture is the Seldinger technique. Several venipuncture techniques have been devised to guide the needle toward the veins (**Table 2**). Venipuncture techniques are possible due to the large diameter of the veins, which can also accommodate multiple leads. This method

Table 2
Summary of the advantages and disadvantages of different axillary and subclavian venipuncture techniques

	Anatomy Only	Fluoroscopy	Contrast Venography	Ultrasound
Advantages	No additional equipment required	Higher success rate	Higher success rate Identifies venous anomalies	Higher success rate No radiation or contrast exposure
Disadvantages	Lower success rates	Radiation exposure to operator and patient	Radiation exposure to operator and patient Risk of contrast allergy and nephropathy	Requires training on ultrasound techniques Most techniques require a second operator

is quicker than cephalic vein cutdown, has a higher success rate, and will leave the leads anatomically closer to the infraclavicular pulse generator site.[3]

As the axillary and subclavian veins form a continuity, the distinction between them may be arbitrary because venipuncture can occur on adjacent venous segments as the needle is advanced medially.[3] Nevertheless, targeting the axillary vein is associated with fewer complications due to its lateral position, which reduces lead stress and the risk of pleural damage. A recent study assigned 247 patients to either axillary or subclavian venipuncture.[15] There were no venipuncture-related complications in the axillary group, whereas the subclavian group had 3 pneumothoraces, although it is unclear whether these differences were statistically significant. The subclavian group had a significantly higher incidence of complications during the perioperative period and follow-ups. Complications included pneumothorax, subclavian crush, lead dislocation, and pocket infection. Success rates were comparable between the 2 groups,[15] which corroborates earlier research.[16]

A disadvantage of using these veins is their close proximity to adjacent arteries, nerves, and the pleural cavity. Therefore, attempts at venipuncture can lead to serious acute complications, such as pneumothorax, hemopneumothorax, brachial plexus injury, phrenic nerve injury, thoracic duct injury, subclavian artery venipuncture, and mechanical damage of the lead.[15,17–19] In a study on subclavian vein access, the most common intraoperative complication was inadvertent arterial puncture (2.7% of subclavian insertions), whereas pneumothoraces occurred in 1.8%.[18]

In the long term, complications of subclavian vein access include fracture of leads, subclavian crush syndrome, and loss of lead insulation.[20–22] Subclavian crush occurs due to the high compression pressures exerted on the lead between the first rib and clavicle, as well as entrapment by ligaments of the subclavius muscle and clavicle.[5–9,20] The risk is strongly associated with multiple lead placement and medial venipuncture, and has a prevalence of up to 7% in the first 5 years after implantation.[7,23]

In contrast to the subclavian vein, axillary vein access is rarely associated with pneumothoraces and brachial plexus injuries.[24] Axillary venipuncture has lower lead complication rates and better efficacy in the long term than the subclavian venous approach.[25] On the other hand, it has a smaller diameter, a more variable anatomic position, and a more lateral position, making it more difficult to puncture.[3] Venous spasm induced by venography-guided axillary venipuncture is an uncommon phenomenon that can produce complete occlusion of the vessel's lumen.[26–28] A recent study of 403 patients who underwent lead insertion via axillary venipuncture observed 12 cases (3%) of axillary vein spasm,[26] although an earlier study reported 8.1% of cases with severe venous spasm. In addition, there has been a report of brachial plexus irritation following axillary vein access.[29]

Patient Positioning During Procedures

The Trendelenburg position can aid venous access by expanding central veins in the upper body, which makes them larger targets and reduces the chance of air embolism. Alternatively, introducing a roll between the scapulae while the patient lies supine moves the shoulders and clavicles posteriorly; this makes it easier for the introducer needle to access the deeper veins.[3]

Exclusively Anatomy-Guided Venipuncture

Using anatomic landmarks to guide infraclavicular venipuncture is the simplest technique to place electrode leads in the subclavian vein. By applying knowledge of the anatomy of the clavicle, ribs, sternum, coracoid process, and deltopectoral groove, the needle can be guided toward the subclavian and axillary veins.[4,30–34] Based on its simple method and low equipment requirements, anatomy-guided approaches were first used for transvenous lead placement. However, this blind approach has fallen out of favor over the years because of the high experience required for reliable venipuncture in comparison with fluoroscopy-guided methods.

Various techniques have been developed, but most rely on identifying the bony landmarks of the shoulder and first rib. A prospective study reviewed contrast venographies and developed surface landmarks for anatomy-guided axillary venipuncture.[35] Ten of 10 patients who underwent venipuncture using these developed landmarks had successful lead placements, whereas access using contrast-guided venipuncture was successful in 9 of 10 cases. It was noted that implantation time was not significantly longer than contrast-guided venipuncture. In addition, it was observed that increasing body mass index positively correlated with fluoroscopic times, time taken for venous access, and contrast volumes used. A larger study developed a novel technique for axillary venipuncture that relies on the cephalic vein as an anatomic landmark.[36] This involved preparing the cephalic vein and advancing a needle 1.5 to 2.0 cm medial and parallel to it to enter the axillary vein. Following attempts in 108 patients, successful cannulation using this new method without fluoroscopy or contrast venography was reported as 92.6%.

Fluoroscopy-Guided Venipuncture

Fluoroscopy can be used to identify bony landmarks in relation to the locations of veins. The axillary vein crosses the first rib just below the inferior border of the clavicle.[37] By fluoroscopically identifying the first rib, the needle can be correctly oriented to minimize the risk of a pneumothorax. As the tip of the needle is advanced, its angle can be manipulated while maintaining its fluoroscopic position over the body of the first rib. One study found a 94.5% success rate when using this method to cannulate the axillary vein, whereas the remaining patients were successfully cannulated following contrast venography.[37] More recently, the use of the body surface of the second rib with fluoroscopic landmarks has been proposed for ICD lead implantation; this method produced a significantly higher success rate (100%) compared with using the outer edge of the first rib (88.7%).[38]

Recently, the use of a combination of posterior-anterior and caudal fluoroscopy has been suggested for performing axillary and subclavian venipuncture.[39,40] This allows for better appreciation of the depth of the needle, venous anatomy, and lung borders. In a report of 1207 cases, a study found a twofold to fivefold lower incidence of pneumothorax compared with previously published complications from procedures relying on the conventional posterior-anterior fluoroscopy.[39]

Contrast Venography–Guided Venipuncture

Fluoroscopy in conjunction with contrast venography is commonly used to guide the venipuncture of the subclavian and axillary veins (**Fig. 2**). Contrast dye is injected via peripheral venous access ipsilateral to the desired vein, allowing the route of the axillary and subclavian veins to be visualized.[41–43] Opacification of the venous system provides a "road map" to guide venipuncture at the rib cage margin and facilitate lateral lead entry, minimizing the risk of

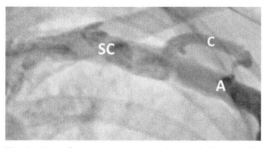

Fig. 2. Use of contrast venography to delineate the course of the cephalic, axillary, and subclavian veins. C, cephalic vein; A, axillary vein; SC, subclavian vein.

subclavian crush injury.[44] In addition, it can reveal anatomic anomalies that may make lead insertion difficult or impossible before attempting venipuncture. In our laboratory, we perform venography before the patient is prepped, which allows for choosing the opposite side if a venous occlusion is present.

A prospective study of axillary vein puncture with or without venography found that venous entry was more likely to be successful with contrast (95%) than without (61%).[42] These high success rates have been corroborated by similar studies, which additionally suggest that the lateral approach provides low rates of complications and lead failure.[11,44–46] A 2016 study compared contrast-guided venipuncture with cephalic cutdown; the success rates between the subclavian (96.8%) and axillary vein (97.6%) were comparable, and were significantly higher than cephalic vein (78.2%). In addition, it was noted that the lowest rates of lead failure were found when using axillary venipuncture.[11]

The limitations of this approach are mainly due to the requirement for contrast dye injection. In comparison with exclusively anatomy-guided venipuncture, ipsilateral peripheral venous access needs to be available. It can trigger an anaphylactic reaction in patients with contrast allergy, which should always be inquired about before the procedure. In our laboratory, patients with contrast allergy are premedicated with Solumedrol and Benadryl if venography is deemed absolutely necessary. In addition, contrast nephropathy is a possible complication, although it is unlikely given the small contrast doses used during the procedure.

Ultrasound-Guided Venipuncture

The use of ultrasound to visualize the needle, vein, and surrounding structures during venipuncture can facilitate lead entry into a lateral position while providing a safe, time-saving method for reducing radiation exposure to the patient and operator, as was first described in 1995.[47] Indeed, central venous access via ultrasound guidance has been highly recommended by the US Agency for Healthcare Research and Quality.[48] Despite its potential advantages, this method has failed to garner much interest until recent years.[49–54]

A recent study reported a 99.25% success rate with no access-related complications when using this method.[51] In comparison with cephalic vein cutdown, ultrasound-guided axillary venous access showed faster lead placement, shorter fluoroscopy times, no differences in the incidence of pocket hematoma or pneumothorax, and comparable success rates.[53] A recent retrospective, single-center study presented the largest analysis of its kind on the outcomes of using the different axillary venipuncture methods. It included 816 patients undergoing cardiac device implantation (137 with ultrasound guidance vs 679 with conventional methods) and concluded that ultrasound-guided vascular access was effective and safe, and complication rates and fluoroscopy times were not significantly lower than traditional methods.[49]

The use of wireless ultrasound transducers for axillary vein cannulation has recently been suggested as a method to make the procedure more effective and safer.[50] This is hypothesized to be due to the easier handling of the probe and lack of need for a second operator. Although the use of wireless transducers was found to be feasible and safe, there have yet to be any randomized studies that compare it to conventional ultrasound or other venipuncture techniques.[50]

UNCOMMON APPROACHES

Although the most commonly used approaches for transvenous lead insertion are through the cephalic, subclavian, or axillary veins, it is not always possible or practical to use these veins.[55–59] Indeed, conventional approaches are contraindicated or impossible in 1% to 6% of patients.[60–63] Such cases can occur with venous obstruction, thrombosis, or fibrosis, as well as variations in cardiovascular anatomy. Several transvenous approaches have been described for pacemaker or defibrillator lead insertion through alternative veins, be it in the upper or lower circulation. Although they are not routinely used as the first choice because of access difficulties, they provide a potential avenue for avoiding epicardial lead placement.

External Jugular Vein

Use of the external jugular vein was initially explored as an option for lead placement, but has failed to gain much attention because of medical and cosmetic reasons.[64,65] In addition, there have been reported cases of pressure necrosis and perforation of the skin of the neck after use of this vein[66]; it has been suggested that this long-term complication could be caused by the sharp angulation of the lead as it enters the vein.

Access can be gained through a cutdown technique in a similar fashion to the cephalic vein. Asking the patient to lie in the Trendelenburg position or perform the Valsalva maneuver can assist in visualizing the course of the external jugular vein.[3] Alternatively, placing a finger above the medial end of the clavicle can engorge it by blocking its venous drainage.[64]

Internal Jugular Vein

Similarly, the use of the internal jugular vein for lead placement has been investigated.[58,67–70] Despite being more amenable to venipuncture because of its large size and deeper location, the use of the internal jugular vein is reserved for cases in which conventional approaches are not possible, such as occlusion or fibrosis.

One study in 2004 recruited 35 patients with occlusion of the upper veins, of which 27 underwent pacemaker or defibrillator lead insertion via cutdown of the internal jugular vein.[58] No intraoperative or perioperative complications were observed. Up to 14 years of follow-up revealed no lead dislodgement, thrombosis, or migration.

Iliofemoral Vein

The femoral vein is the continuation of the popliteal vein and begins at the adductor canal. Once it passes superior to the inguinal ligament, it drains into the external iliac vein. Venipuncture of the iliac or femoral vein can be used to introduce leads into the heart via the inferior vena cava. For the purposes of this review, the iliac and femoral vein approaches are discussed together, as studies use the terms interchangeably because of their close proximity and the distinction may be artificial. Indeed, Ellestad and French[63] corrected the terminology used in their later papers when it came to their attention that the lead enters the vein above the inguinal ligament, so should have been termed the iliac rather than femoral vein.

A recent study analyzed 10-year outcomes of 50 patients undergoing femoral venipuncture.[1] Results showed no major complications at 10-year follow-up, and outcomes were comparable to implantation via the superior venous approach. Elayi and colleagues[71] developed a novel approach, the inside-out central venous access, which uses the femoral vein to puncture occluded central venous segments before advancing the needle to exit the body, providing a new channel for transvenous lead implantation. All 8 patients with central venous occlusions who underwent this new approach had successful device implantations with no procedure-related complications.

In recent years, there have been successful cases reporting use of the iliofemoral approach due to upper circulation occlusion or variations in anatomy.[1,55,56,59–61,63,71–74] Several studies have observed a high rate of atrial lead displacement in the long term.[61,63] Analysis of the outcomes of 27 patients with femoral pacemakers showed that atrial lead displacement occurred in 20% of cases.[61] Another consideration when using the iliofemoral approach is the requirement for specific long leads, which are more difficult to manipulate. Nevertheless, more recent research showed outcomes were comparable to superior venous lead insertion with low rates of atrial lead displacement.[1,73]

Supraclavicular Subclavian Vein

Although the infraclavicular approach is most commonly used in clinical practice for subclavian venipuncture, venous obstruction of the vessel can complicate this procedure. Therefore, a supraclavicular route can be successful if leads are inserted proximal to the occlusion site. Liu and colleagues[75] used this method for 44 patients and, in comparison with an infraclavicular approach, reported faster venipuncture times but slightly more blood loss. No lead dislodgement, lead fracture, or skin erosion were encountered. Similar results have been found in other studies,[76,77] which suggests that this alternative approach can be safely used in cases of venous obstruction.

Brachiocephalic Vein

A lateral infraclavicular approach can be used to gain access to the brachiocephalic vein. A 2014 study used this technique on 14 patients with subclavian and cephalic vein occlusion.[78] All 14 were successful and without complications, notably pneumothoraces. Follow-up (mean 36 weeks) showed no evidence of lead failure or impedance changes, and all implanted leads were functioning well.

Supraclavicular percutaneous access is an alternative approach for brachiocephalic access. Ovadia and colleagues[79] used this in 5 pediatric patients and 1 adult patient with subclavian vein obstruction, which were successful and without any complications.

Azygos Vein

Directly accessing the azygos vein for transvenous lead insertion is an invasive procedure that has been described for a patient with superior vena cava syndrome[57]: a 73-year-old patient who had bilateral occlusion of the subclavian veins following previous bilateral pectoral pacemaker implantation via the subclavian vein. The azygos vein was dissected and accessed by performing right lateral minimal thoracotomy while the patient was in a left lateral decubitus position. Follow-up revealed that electrode placement was stable and the patient was symptom-free with normal pacemaker function for 1.5 years.

SPECIAL CONSIDERATION: PERSISTENT LEFT SUPERIOR VENA CAVA

A persistent left superior vena cava (PLSVC) is the most common venous anomaly of the thorax[80] that occurs following failure of embryologic obliteration of the left anterior cardinal vein[81,82] (**Fig. 3**). Of candidates for pacemaker insertion or cardioverter-defibrillator implantation, 0.3% to 2.0% have PLSVC,[81] which is comparable to the general population.[83] Most cases are asymptomatic, although it is associated with a 10-fold higher

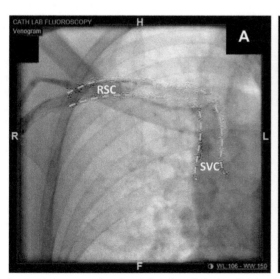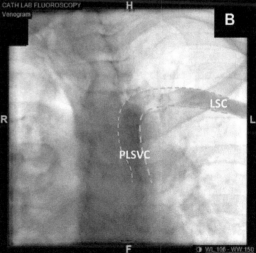

Fig. 3. Venograms showing (*A*) right subclavian (RSC) vein draining into superior vena cava (SVC); (*B*) left subclavian (LSC) draining into a PLSVC in the same patient; there was no bridging vein between SVC and PLSVC as is sometimes present.

incidence in congenital heart disease[83,84]; indeed, 3% to 10% of patients with congenital heart disease are found to have a PLSVC.[85] Therefore, it usually remains unrecognized and incidentally discovered when transcatheter approaches are attempted via the cephalic or subclavian veins.

Lead implantation via a PLSVC can be technically difficult, and sometimes impossible.[81,83,86,87] This is due to unfavorable anatomy and limited availability of suitable leads.[82,84] The major difficulty is deflection of the lead's tip away from the tricuspid annulus during right ventricular implantation,[86] which can prolong radiation and procedure times.[85] In the long term, the loop on the lead across the tricuspid valve can undergo higher mechanical stress and consequent lead failure.[85] One study found that PLSVC does not influence pacing parameters in the long term.[88] Given these difficulties, some operators opt for an approach on the right side once a PLSVC is identified.

Nevertheless, there have been numerous reports of successful implantations via the left or right subclavian veins.[80,83,84,86,89] A case series on 5 PLSVC patients revealed that the long-term outcome following transvenous lead implantation was mostly influenced by underlying heart disease.[86] In some cases, a small branch communicating between the PLSVC and right superior vena cava can be used to gain entry to the brachiocephalic vein and superior vena cava.[85] Communicating branches between the PLSVC and right-sided venous drainage may be found in 50% of PLSVC cases.[85,90]

FUTURE DIRECTIONS

The increasing demand for permanent pacemaker and ICD implantations with an aging population necessitates the exploration and refinement of transvenous approaches to deal with the consequent rise in complications. The use of ultrasound-guided venipuncture has begun to be investigated with promising safety and efficacy results, although it has yet to experience widespread use. In recent years, leadless pacemaker systems have been developed that provide an avenue for circumventing the inherent complications of conventional pacemakers, although only single-chamber stimulation is currently available and their clinical efficacy is yet to be fully elucidated with long-term, randomized clinical trials.[91,92]

SUMMARY

Transvenous approaches for pacemaker and defibrillator lead insertion offer numerous advantages over epicardial techniques. Although the cephalic,

axillary, and subclavian veins are most commonly used in clinical practice, they each offer their own set of advantages and disadvantages that leave their usage dependent on patient anatomy and physician preference. Alternative methods using the upper and lower venous circulation have been described when these veins are not available or practical for lead insertion. Until current technology is superseded by leadless pacing systems, the search for the optimal lead insertion technique continues.

REFERENCES

1. Garcia Guerrero JJ, Fernandez de la Concha Castaneda J, Doblado Calatrava M, et al. Transfemoral access when superior venous approach is not feasible equals overall success of permanent pacemaker implantation. Ten-year series. Pacing Clin Electrophysiol 2017;40(6):638–43.
2. Bongiorni MG, Proclemer A, Dobreanu D, et al. Preferred tools and techniques for implantation of cardiac electronic devices in Europe: results of the European Heart Rhythm Association survey. Europace 2013;15(11):1664–8.
3. Lau EW. Upper body venous access for transvenous lead placement–review of existent techniques. Pacing Clin Electrophysiol 2007;30(7):901–9.
4. Jaques PF, Campbell WE, Dumbleton S, et al. The first rib as a fluoroscopic marker for subclavian vein access. J Vasc Interv Radiol 1995;6(4):619–22.
5. Paiva L, Providencia R, Faustino A, et al. Subclavian crush syndrome and subcutaneous ICD in primary prevention patients. J Cardiovasc Med (Hagerstown) 2017;18(9):717–8.
6. Femenia F, Diez JC, Arce M, et al. Subclavian crush syndrome: a cause of pacemaker lead fracture. Cardiovasc J Afr 2011;22(4):201–2.
7. Gallik DM, Ben-Zur UM, Gross JN, et al. Lead fracture in cephalic versus subclavian approach with transvenous implantable cardioverter defibrillator systems. Pacing Clin Electrophysiol 1996;19(7):1089–94.
8. Roelke M, O'Nunain SS, Osswald S, et al. Subclavian crush syndrome complicating transvenous cardioverter defibrillator systems. Pacing Clin Electrophysiol 1995;18(5 Pt 1):973–9.
9. Magney JE, Flynn DM, Parsons JA, et al. Anatomical mechanisms explaining damage to pacemaker leads, defibrillator leads, and failure of central venous catheters adjacent to the sternoclavicular joint. Pacing Clin Electrophysiol 1993;16(3 Pt 1):445–57.
10. Kolettis TM, Lysitsas DN, Apostolidis D, et al. Improved 'cut-down' technique for transvenous pacemaker lead implantation. Europace 2010;12(9):1282–5.

11. Chan NY, Kwong NP, Cheong AP. Venous access and long-term pacemaker lead failure: comparing contrast-guided axillary vein puncture with subclavian puncture and cephalic cutdown. Europace 2017;19(7):1193–7.

12. Neri R, Cesario AS, Baragli D, et al. Permanent pacing lead insertion through the cephalic vein using an hydrophilic guidewire. Pacing Clin Electrophysiol 2003;26(12):2313–4.

13. Calkins H, Ramza BM, Brinker J, et al. Prospective randomized comparison of the safety and effectiveness of placement of endocardial pacemaker and defibrillator leads using the extrathoracic subclavian vein guided by contrast venography versus the cephalic approach. Pacing Clin Electrophysiol 2001; 24(4 Pt 1):456–64.

14. Tse HF, Lau CP, Leung SK. A cephalic vein cutdown and venography technique to facilitate pacemaker and defibrillator lead implantation. Pacing Clin Electrophysiol 2001;24(4 Pt 1):469–73.

15. Liu P, Zhou YF, Yang P, et al. Optimized axillary vein technique versus subclavian vein technique in cardiovascular implantable electronic device implantation: a randomized controlled study. Chin Med J (Engl) 2016;129(22):2647–51.

16. Sharma G, Senguttuvan NB, Thachil A, et al. A comparison of lead placement through the subclavian vein technique with fluoroscopy-guided axillary vein technique for permanent pacemaker insertion. Can J Cardiol 2012;28(5):542–6.

17. Tobin K, Stewart J, Westveer D, et al. Acute complications of permanent pacemaker implantation: their financial implication and relation to volume and operator experience. Am J Cardiol 2000;85(6):774–6. A779.

18. Aggarwal RK, Connelly DT, Ray SG, et al. Early complications of permanent pacemaker implantation: no difference between dual and single chamber systems. Br Heart J 1995;73(6):571–5.

19. Chauhan A, Grace AA, Newell SA, et al. Early complications after dual chamber versus single chamber pacemaker implantation. Pacing Clin Electrophysiol 1994;17(11 Pt 2):2012–5.

20. Antonelli D, Rosenfeld T, Freedberg NA, et al. Insulation lead failure: is it a matter of insulation coating, venous approach, or both? Pacing Clin Electrophysiol 1998;21(2):418–21.

21. Kazama S, Nishiyama K, Machii M, et al. Long-term follow up of ventricular endocardial pacing leads. Complications, electrical performance, and longevity of 561 right ventricular leads. Jpn Heart J 1993;34(2): 193–200.

22. Alt E, Volker R, Blomer H. Lead fracture in pacemaker patients. Thorac Cardiovasc Surg 1987; 35(2):101–4.

23. Migliore F, Curnis A, Bertaglia E. Axillary vein technique for pacemaker and implantable defibrillator leads implantation: a safe and alternative approach? J Cardiovasc Med (Hagerstown) 2016;17(4):309–13.

24. Hess DS, Gertz EW, Morady F, et al. Permanent pacemaker implantation in the cardiac catheterization laboratory: the subclavian vein approach. Cathet Cardiovasc Diagn 1982;8(5):453–8.

25. Kim KH, Park KM, Nam GB, et al. Comparison of the axillary venous approach and subclavian venous approach for efficacy of permanent pacemaker implantation. 8-Year follow-up results. Circ J 2014; 78(4):865–71.

26. Steckiewicz R, Gorko D, Swieton EB, et al. Axillary vein spasm during cardiac implantable electronic device implantation. Folia Morphol 2016;75(4):543–9.

27. Duan X, Ling F, Shen Y, et al. Venous spasm during contrast-guided axillary vein puncture for pacemaker or defibrillator lead implantation. Europace 2012;14(7):1008–11.

28. Chan NY, Leung WS. Venospasm in contrast venography-guided axillary vein puncture for pacemaker lead implantation. Pacing Clin Electrophysiol 2003;26(1 Pt 1):112–3.

29. Kim SY, Park JS, Bang JH, et al. Brachial plexus injury caused by indwelling axillary venous pacing leads. Korean Circ J 2015;45(5):428–31.

30. Belott PH. Blind axillar venous access. Pacing Clin Electrophysiol 1999;22(7):1085–9.

31. Magney JE, Staplin DH, Flynn DM, et al. A new approach to percutaneous subclavian venipuncture to avoid lead fracture or central venous catheter occlusion. Pacing Clin Electrophysiol 1993;16(11): 2133–42.

32. Taylor BL, Yellowlees I. Central venous cannulation using the infraclavicular axillary vein. Anesthesiology 1990;72(1):55–8.

33. Nickalls RW. A new percutaneous infraclavicular approach to the axillary vein. Anaesthesia 1987; 42(2):151–4.

34. Borja AR, Hinshaw JR. A safe way to perform infraclavicular subclavian vein catheterization. Surg Gynecol Obstet 1970;130(4):673–6.

35. Mehrotra S, Rohit MK. Prospective study to develop surface landmarks for blind axillary vein puncture for permanent pacemaker and defibrillator lead implantation and compare it to available contrast venography guided technique. Indian Heart J 2015; 67(2):136–40.

36. Imnadze G, Awad K, Wolff E, et al. A novel method of axillary venipuncture using the cephalic vein as a sole anatomic landmark. Can J Cardiol 2015; 31(8):1067–9.

37. Antonelli D, Feldman A, Freedberg NA, et al. Axillary vein puncture without contrast venography for pacemaker and defibrillator leads implantation. Pacing Clin Electrophysiol 2013;36(9):1107–10.

38. Migliore F, Siciliano M, De Lazzari M, et al. Axillary vein puncture using fluoroscopic landmarks: a safe

and effective approach for implantable cardioverter defibrillator leads. J Interv Card Electrophysiol 2015; 43(3):263–7.

39. Patel HC, Hayward C, Nanayakkara S, et al. Caudal fluoroscopy to guide venous access for pacemaker device implantation: should this now be standard practice? Heart Asia 2017;9(1):68–9.

40. Yang F, Kulbak G. A new trick to a routine procedure: taking the fear out of the axillary vein stick using the 35 degrees caudal view. Europace 2015;17(7): 1157–60.

41. Belott P. How to access the axillary vein. Heart Rhythm 2006;3(3):366–9.

42. Burri H, Sunthorn H, Dorsaz PA, et al. Prospective study of axillary vein puncture with or without contrast venography for pacemaker and defibrillator lead implantation. Pacing Clin Electrophysiol 2005; 28(Suppl 1):S280–3.

43. Byrd CL. Safe introducer technique for pacemaker lead implantation. Pacing Clin Electrophysiol 1992; 15(3):262–7.

44. Spencer WH 3rd, Zhu DW, Kirkpatrick C, et al. Subclavian venogram as a guide to lead implantation. Pacing Clin Electrophysiol 1998;21(3):499–502.

45. Harada Y, Katsume A, Kimata M, et al. Placement of pacemaker leads via the extrathoracic subclavian vein guided by fluoroscopy and venography in the oblique projection. Heart Vessels 2005;20(1):19–22.

46. Dora SK, Kumar VK, Bhat A, et al. Venogram-guided extrathoracic subclavian vein puncture. Indian Heart J 2003;55(6):637–40.

47. Fyke FE 3rd. Doppler guided extrathoracic introducer insertion. Pacing Clin Electrophysiol 1995; 18(5 Pt 1):1017–21.

48. Shekelle PG, Wachter RM, Pronovost PJ, et al. Making health care safer II: an updated critical analysis of the evidence for patient safety practices. Evid Rep Technol Assess (Full Rep) 2013;(211):1–945.

49. Lin J, Adsit G, Barnett A, et al. Feasibility of ultrasound-guided vascular access during cardiac implantable device placement. J Interv Card Electrophysiol 2017;50(1):105–9.

50. Franco E, Rodriguez Munoz D, Matia R, et al. Wireless ultrasound-guided axillary vein cannulation for the implantation of cardiovascular implantable electric devices. J Cardiovasc Electrophysiol 2016; 27(4):482–7.

51. Esmaiel A, Hassan J, Blenkhorn F, et al. The use of ultrasound to improve axillary vein access and minimize complications during pacemaker implantation. Pacing Clin Electrophysiol 2016;39(5):478–82.

52. Seto AH, Jolly A, Salcedo J. Ultrasound-guided venous access for pacemakers and defibrillators. J Cardiovasc Electrophysiol 2013;24(3):370–4.

53. Jones DG, Stiles MK, Stewart JT, et al. Ultrasound-guided venous access for permanent pacemaker leads. Pacing Clin Electrophysiol 2006;29(8):852–7.

54. Orihashi K, Imai K, Sato K, et al. Extrathoracic subclavian venipuncture under ultrasound guidance. Circ J 2005;69(9):1111–5.

55. Agosti S, Brunelli C, Bertero G. Biventricular pacemaker implantation via the femoral vein. J Clin Med Res 2012;4(4):289–91.

56. Dhillon PS, Gallagher MM. Femoral vein implantation with subclavian vein pullthrough for left ventricular lead placement. Europace 2010;12(8):1193–4.

57. Goktekin O, Besoglu Y, Dogan SM, et al. Permanent pacemaker lead implantation via azygous vein in a patient with silent superior vena cava syndrome. Int J Cardiol 2007;117(1). e4–6.

58. Molina JE. Surgical options for endocardial lead placement when upper veins are obstructed or nonusable. J Interv Card Electrophysiol 2004;11(2):149–54.

59. Perzanowski C, Timothy P, McAfee M, et al. Implantation of implantable cardioverter-defibrillators from an ileofemoral approach. J Interv Card Electrophysiol 2004;11(2):155–9.

60. Yamaguchi T, Miyamoto T, Yamauchi Y, et al. A case report of successful permanent pacemaker implantation via the iliac vein. J Arrhythm 2016;32(2):151–3.

61. Mathur G, Stables RH, Heaven D, et al. Permanent pacemaker implantation via the femoral vein: an alternative in cases with contraindications to the pectoral approach. Europace 2001;3(1):56–9.

62. Barakat K, Hill J, Kelly P. Permanent transfemoral pacemaker implantation is the technique of choice for patients in whom the superior vena cava is inaccessible. Pacing Clin Electrophysiol 2000;23(4 Pt 1):446–9.

63. Ellestad MH, French J. Iliac vein approach to permanent pacemaker implantation. Pacing Clin Electrophysiol 1989;12(7 Pt 1):1030–3.

64. Furman S. Venous cutdown for pacemaker implantation. Ann Thorac Surg 1986;41(4):438–9.

65. Kemler RL. A simple method for exposing the external jugular vein for placement of a permanent transvenous pacing catheter electrode. Ann Thorac Surg 1978;26(3):266–8.

66. Laforet EG, Rubenstein JJ. Late perforation by pacemaker catheter loop in the neck: a preventable complication of the external jugular approach. South Med J 1986;79(3):384–5.

67. Molina JE, Dunnigan AC, Crosson JE. Implantation of transvenous pacemakers in infants and small children. Ann Thorac Surg 1995;59(3):689–94.

68. Brodman R, Furman S. Pacemaker implantation through the internal jugular vein. Ann Thorac Surg 1980;29(1):63–5.

69. Rao G, Zikria EA. Technique of insertion of pacing electrode through the internal jugular vein. J Cardiovasc Surg (Torino) 1973;14(3):294.

70. Leininger BJ, Neville WE. Use of the internal jugular vein for implantations of permanent transvenous pacemakers. Experiences with 22 patients. Ann Thorac Surg 1968;5(1):61–5.

71. Elayi CS, Allen CL, Leung S, et al. Inside-out access: a new method of lead placement for patients with central venous occlusions. Heart Rhythm 2011; 8(6):851–7.

72. Chaggar PS, Skene C, Williams SG. The transfemoral approach for cardiac resynchronization therapy. Europace 2015;17(2):173.

73. Ching CK, Elayi CS, Di Biase L, et al. Transiliac ICD implantation: defibrillation vector flexibility produces consistent success. Heart Rhythm 2009;6(7):978–83.

74. Antonelli D, Freedberg NA, Rosenfeld T. Transiliac vein approach to a rate responsive permanent pacemaker implantation. Pacing Clin Electrophysiol 1993;16(8):1751–2.

75. Liu KS, Liu C, Xia Y, et al. Permanent cardiac pacing through the right supraclavicular subclavian vein approach. Can J Cardiol 2003;19(9):1005–8.

76. Antonelli D, Freedberg NA, Turgeman Y. Supraclavicular vein approach to overcoming ipsilateral chronic subclavian vein obstruction during pacemaker-ICD lead revision or upgrading. Europace 2010;12(11): 1596–9.

77. Antonelli D, Freedberg NA, Rosenfeld T. Lead insertion by supraclavicular approach of the subclavian vein puncture. Pacing Clin Electrophysiol 2001; 24(3):379–80.

78. Bernstein NE, Aizer A, Chinitz LA. Use of a lateral infraclavicular puncture to obtain proximal venous access with occluded subclavian/axillary venous systems for cardiac rhythm devices. Pacing Clin Electrophysiol 2014;37(8):1017–22.

79. Ovadia M, Cooper RS, Parnell VA, et al. Transvenous pacemaker insertion ipsilateral to chronic subclavian vein obstruction: an operative technique for children and adults. Pacing Clin Electrophysiol 2000;23(11 Pt 1):1585–93.

80. Bissinger A, Bahadori-Esfahani F, Lubinski A. Cardiac defibrillator implantation via persistent left superior vena cava—sometimes this approach is facile. A case report. Arch Med Sci 2011;7(1):161–3.

81. Ratliff HL, Yousufuddin M, Lieving WR, et al. Persistent left superior vena cava: case reports and clinical implications. Int J Cardiol 2006;113(2):242–6.

82. Polewczyk A, Kutarski A, Czekajska-Chehab E, et al. Complications of permanent cardiac pacing in patients with persistent left superior vena cava. Cardiol J 2014;21(2):128–37.

83. Biffi M, Bertini M, Ziacchi M, et al. Clinical implications of left superior vena cava persistence in candidates for pacemaker or cardioverter-defibrillator implantation. Heart Vessels 2009;24(2):142–6.

84. Guenther M, Kolschmann S, Rauwolf TP, et al. Implantable cardioverter defibrillator lead implantation in patients with a persistent left superior vena cava–feasibility, chances, and limitations: representative cases in adults. Europace 2013;15(2):273–7.

85. Kumar V, Yoshida N, Yamada T. Successful implantable cardioverter-defibrillator implantation through a communicating branch of the persistent left superior vena cava. J arrhythmia 2015;31(5):331–2.

86. Petrac D, Radeljic V, Pavlovic N, et al. Persistent left superior vena cava in patients undergoing cardiac device implantation: clinical and long-term data. Cardiol Res 2013;4(2):64–7.

87. Fischer S, Hofs T. Persistent left superior vena cava as a cause for an unsuccessful ICD implant. Herzschrittmacherther Elektrophysiol 2009;20(1):43–6.

88. Dabrowski P, Obszanski B, Kleinrok A, et al. Long-term follow-up after pacemaker implantation via persistent left superior vena cava. Cardiol J 2014; 21(4):413–8.

89. Jovic Z, Mijailovic Z, Obradovic S, et al. Successful implantation of a permanent pacemaker through a persistent left superior vena cava by using a right subclavian approach. Vojnosanit Pregl 2011;68(9): 792–4.

90. Peltier J, Destrieux C, Desme J, et al. The persistent left superior vena cava: anatomical study, pathogenesis and clinical considerations. Surg Radiol Anat 2006;28(2):206–10.

91. Merkel M, Grotherr P, Radzewitz A, et al. Leadless pacing: current state and future direction. Cardiol Ther 2017;6(2):175–81.

92. Miller MA, Neuzil P, Dukkipati SR, et al. Leadless cardiac pacemakers: back to the future. J Am Coll Cardiol 2015;66(10):1179–89.

Monitoring for and Diagnosis of Lead Dysfunction

Sandeep G. Nair, MD[1], Charles D. Swerdlow, MD*

KEYWORDS

- Implantable cardioverter-defibrillator • Pacemaker • Lead dysfunction • Lead failure

KEY POINTS

- The predominant structural mechanisms of transvenous lead dysfunction (LD) are conductor fracture and insulation breach.
- LD typically presents as an abnormality of electrical performance; the earliest sign usually is oversensing or out-of-range pacing or shock impedance.
- Accurate diagnosis of LD requires discriminating patterns of oversensing and impedance trends that are characteristic of LD from similar patterns that occur in other conditions.
- Implantable cardioverter-defibrillators have advanced features to detect and mitigate the consequences of LD; these features operate both independently and in conjunction with remote monitoring networks.

All mechanical components have finite service lives. Transvenous leads of cardiac implantable electronic device (CIED) systems are expected to operate for decades in a chemically hostile environment, subject to multiple mechanical stresses.[1] Despite advances in design, bench testing, and clinical testing, structural elements of leads fail during clinical service, often with serious clinical consequences. Monitoring for and accurate diagnosis of lead dysfunction (LD) is thus an essential element of the cardiac electrophysiologist's tool kit.

This review focuses on LD of multilumen, transvenous, right ventricular (RV), implantable cardioverter-defibrillator (ICD) leads because they have a higher failure rate than pacing leads. Most aspects of monitoring and diagnosis for pace-sense elements of ICD leads apply with minor modifications to pacing leads, which are mentioned briefly. We assume basic knowledge of the design, components, and construction of coaxial, multilumen, and coradial transvenous leads.[2,3]

DEFINITIONS

We use LD to mean *mechanical LD*, defined as failure of one or more lead structural elements, and *electrical LD* to mean mechanical LD that causes abnormal electrical performance. This includes failure to perform the lead's clinically intended electrical function (sensing, pacing, or defibrillation), unintended stimulation of noncardiac muscle, or out-of-range values for clinically measured, lead-related electrical parameters (eg, impedance). In this construct, electrical LD does not occur without preexisting mechanical LD, but mechanical LD does not necessarily cause electrical LD. For example, in multilumen defibrillation leads, silicone inside-out, mechanical insulation

Disclosures: The authors have nothing to disclose.
Cedars Sinai Heart Institute, 8700 Beverly Boulevard, Los Angeles, CA 90048, USA
[1] Present address: 400 South Burnside Avenue, Apartment 1M, Los Angeles, CA.
* Corresponding author. 414 North Camden Drive, Suite 1100, Beverly Hills, CA 90210.
E-mail address: swerdlow@g.ucla.edu

Card Electrophysiol Clin 10 (2018) 573–599
https://doi.org/10.1016/j.ccep.2018.07.004

cardiacEP.theclinics.com

breaches[4] often occur without electrical LD, providing that inner ethylene tetrafluoroethylene (ETFE) insulation remains intact surrounding each cable.[5] We do not address failure of the lead to perform its clinical role in the absence of mechanical LD (*functional LD*), such as intracavitary dislodgement,[6] microscopic dislodgement ("microdislodgement"),[7] chamber-wall perforation, or electrode-myocardial interface issues.[8] Clinically diagnosed LD is caused almost exclusively by electrical LD. Rare exceptions include damage to the tricuspid valve or other structures caused by externalized cables in inside-out insulation breaches.

CLASSIFICATION OF LEAD DYSFUNCTION

It is useful to classify LD mechanically, by the structural element that fails. Clinically, however, we work backward from manifestations of electrical LD, including clinical consequences and changes in device electrograms (EGMs) or automated diagnostics, to the root, structural failure.

Mechanical Lead Dysfunction: Classification by Structural Element

The vast majority of LD is caused by either conductor fracture or insulation breach.

Conductor fracture

Conductor fractures are caused by mechanical stress. Low-cycle, high-load forces near the vein insertion site usually fracture the helix to the tip electrode. High-cycle, low-load forces caused by cardiac motion usually fracture the cable to the ring electrode of dedicated bipolar leads. Shock conductors may fracture at multiple locations.[9] Conductor fractures usually involve either pace-sense (low-voltage) or shock (high-voltage) conductors; simultaneous failures of multiple conductors are uncommon.

Insulation breach

Most insulation breaches are caused by abrasion and cold flow ("creep") of silicone or chemical degradation of polyurethane. The most common cause of insulation breach is external ("outside-in"), caused by abrasion or compressive forces between the lead and pacemaker/defibrillator can or between 2 leads. Less common internal ("inside-out") abrasion of multilumen leads is caused by cyclical forces exerted by lead cables on silicone insulation[4] (the pace-sense cable to the ring electrode, the shock cable to the RV coil, and or shock cable to the superior vena cava [SVC] coil). They often result in complete abrasion of insulation between 2 conductors. In contrast, outside-in insulation breaches usually expose one conductor to extracellular fluid, although extensive abrasion can expose multiple conductors. Insulation breaches of the central, helical conductor to the tip electrode require sufficient external, localized force to cause multiple lead elements to fail (**Fig. 1**). This may occur with subclavian crush[10] or localized anchor-sleeve damage[11] (**Fig. 2**).

In coaxial pacemaker leads, outside-in abrasion exposes the helix to the ring electrode. Chemical, metal-ion oxidative degradation[12] of inner polyurethane insulation can cause a breach that shorts the outer helix to the inner helix.

Correlation Between Mechanical and Electrical Lead Dysfunction

Basic concepts

- *Conductor fractures interrupt therapeutic current pathways*, either completely or partially. Interruption is usually intermittent. Partial conductor fractures are often subclinical. Electrical LD may be caused by failure to conduct sensed cardiac signals to the generator, failure to conduct therapeutic pacing or defibrillation pulses from the generator to the heart, and, most commonly, by generation of abnormal signals. These signals often are referred to as "make-break" potentials because indistinguishable signals can be generated by connecting and disconnecting cables from the sensing circuit[13] and because it is surmised that a similar process applies during intermittent contact between fractured sections of conductors.[2] However, it is uncertain if the make-break mechanism explains pacing-induced signals related to conductor fractures.[14]

- In contrast, *insulation breaches open an alternate, parallel pathway for current flow* into and out of conductors. The nature of electrical LD depends on the relative electrical impedances of the parallel and primary pathways. Usually, the impedance of the parallel pathway is higher than the impedance of pacing pathways and more than 10 times higher than the impedance of shock pathways. Such breaches have little effect on the amplitude of sensed EGMs, or pacing capture from constant-voltage CIED sources. Unlike conductor fractures, insulation breaches themselves are not sources of abnormal signals, but abnormal signals may enter the intact conductor at the breach. Hence, pace-sense insulation breaches present

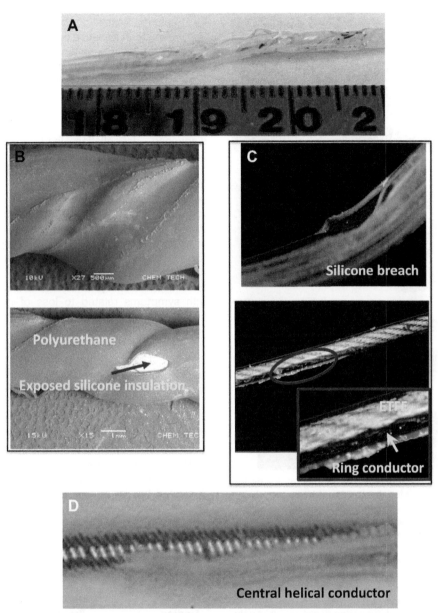

Fig. 1. Outside-in, insulation breach involving multiple insulation layers and multiple conductors occurring below the clavicle in a Medtronic Quattro 6947M lead. **Fig. 7** displays corresponding oversensing events and impedance trend. (*A*) Optical image of intact lead (after extraction), showing twisted and deformed outer polyurethane insulation. (*B*) Scanning electron micrographs of intact lead (before destructive analysis). Upper panel provides more detailed image of twisted and deformed outer polyurethane insulation. Lower panel shows polyurethane insulation breach, exposing inner silicone insulation tubing. (*C*) Scanning electron micrographs show destructive analysis of lead. Upper panel shows breach in silicone tubing. The breach appeared as a slit when the tubing was straight, but became a gap when the lead was bent in compression, simulating subclavian crush. Lower panel shows inner ETFE insulation breach on conductor to ring electrode seen in the panel insert at lower right. (*D*) Further destructive analysis exposed central helical conductor, showing extensive breach of its layer of inner ETFE insulation. Most outside-in insulation breaches expose cables but do not reach the inner coil of multilumen leads. (*Courtesy of* Medtronic, Inc., Minneapolis, MN. © Medtronic 2018.)

most commonly as a result of signals from external sources entering the affected conductor(s). However, when the impedance of the parallel pathway is less than the impedance of the primary pathway, insulation breaches may interfere with sensing and pacing. Further, high-voltage breaches may have high impedance when measured with

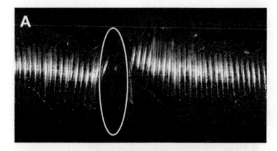

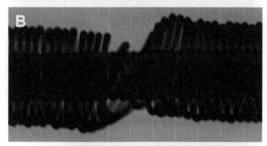

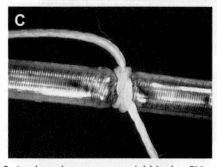

Fig. 2. Implant damage to coaxial bipolar, RV pacing lead (Biotronik Model 377176) with outer polyurethane and inner silicone insulation breach, in a patient with complete heart block. When a suture sleeve was tightened on the anchor sleeve, there was no pacing capture at maximum output and the measured bipolar impedance was less than 100 Ω. When the suture was cut, the pacing threshold returned to baseline and impedance returned to nominal. Inspection showed that the anchor sleeve split at the suture site. (*A*) Optical photo shows the deformation (*yellow oval*) of polyurethane insulation and outer pacing coil to ring electrode. (*B*) Radiograph shows permanent deformation of outer pacing coil without fracture. Electrical testing confirmed that both inner and outer coils had electrical continuity; impedance remained constant during aggressive manipulation around the damage site. (*C*) Optical image shows no silicone insulation breach. A suture fits precisely into the depression in the insulation. (*Courtesy of* Biotronik, Inc, Berlin, Germany.)

low-amplitude diagnostic pulses (and hence go undetected), but extremely low impedance during a defibrillation shock, diverting the shock from the heart. Like conductor

fractures, insulation breaches are usually intermittent, because conductors have multiple redundant layers of insulation and deformed silicone partially returns to its original shape after the applied force is removed.

Device function affected

Pace-sense LDs account for most clinically diagnosed defibrillation lead failures[15] and present most commonly as the result of oversensing the related abnormal signals: alerts from device diagnostics triggered by oversensing[16–18] or inappropriate detection of ventricular tachycardia (VT) or fibrillation (VF), either asymptomatic nonsustained episodes or sustained episodes resulting in inappropriate shocks.[8,17,19–22] Pace-sense failure in pacemaker-dependent patients with either defibrillation or pacing leads commonly presents with symptoms related to loss of pacing (**Table 1**). In patients with an escape rhythm, pace-sense failure may present with undersensing due to abrupt decrease in R-wave amplitude.[15–17] Less common failures of high-voltage components result in failure to deliver therapeutic shocks.

Symptoms

Most symptoms of electrical LD neither distinguish LD from other causes of electrical abnormalities nor discriminate among mechanisms of LD. However, pectoral muscle stimulation by a dedicated bipolar pacing is diagnostic of an in-pocket insulation breach, providing retraction of

Table 1
Electrical manifestations of lead dysfunction

Finding	Insulation Breach	Conductor Fracture
Increased pacing impedance	—	X
Decreased pacing impedance	X	—
Increased high-voltage coil impedance	—	X
Oversensing[a]	X	X
Undersensing	X	—
Myopotential	X	—
Failure to capture	X	X
Failure to defibrillate	X	X

[a] Including inappropriate shocks and failure to pace.

the lead tip to the pocket is excluded by chest radiograph.

Time course of lead dysfunction

Most LD presents late after lead implant, almost always more than 6 months, more commonly years.[23] However, intraoperative damage at lead implant or generator change may present perioperatively. Intraoperative damage includes insulation breaches caused by surgical instruments or electrocautery, insulation breaches or conductor fracture due to anchor-sleeve sutures (see **Fig. 2**), or damage to the retractable screw of an active fixation lead.[3]

PRIMARY DIAGNOSTIC TOOLS

Cardiac Implantable Electronic Device Electrograms

Because oversensing is the most common abnormality in pace-sense LD, device EGMs, together with their corresponding interval and episode data, play a central role in diagnosis.

Principles of electrogram interpretation for diagnosis of lead dysfunction

- For dedicated bipolar ICD leads, signals on the sensing channel that do not correspond to the signals on the shock channel indicate oversensing.[24] Thus, the shock EGM serves as a check on the sensing EGM in determining whether signals on the sensing EGM represent ventricular depolarization.
- *Stored EGMs* from device-detected tachycardias and device-classified oversensing events are primary sources for evaluating LD-related oversensing.
- *Real-time EGMs* recorded in clinic during various physical maneuvers (**Table 2**) may provoke both LD-related oversensing caused by in-pocket structural failures (**Fig. 3**) and specific, non–LD-related mechanisms of oversensing. See details later in this article.
- *Differential EGMs* recorded simultaneously between 1 common electrode and 2 different electrodes can determine the conductor(s) involved in oversensing, when stored EGMs provide insufficient information[2] (see **Fig. 3**). Knowing the involved conductors facilitates management if this conductor can be removed from the pace-sense or defibrillation pathway, either temporarily or permanently.
- *The temporal pattern of oversensed signals may facilitate diagnosis of LD-related oversensing.* Oversensing may vary with the ventricular cycle (*cyclical*, **Fig. 4**) or independently of the ventricular cycle (*noncyclical*, see **Fig. 3**; **Fig. 5**). Cyclical

Table 2 Physical maneuvers for the diagnosis of lead dysfunction	
Physical Maneuver	**What to Look for**
Stretching and isometric exercise (hands clasped pulling against each other, palm of both hands pushing against each other, reaching right shoulder with left arm and left shoulder with right arm, pectoral muscle exercise).	Noncardiac signals on sensing channel. Myopotentials are a normal finding on intact shock channels, but transient high-frequency signals may occur with shock coil fractures at vein insertion site or under clavicle (subclavian crush).
Device pocket manipulation.	Oversensing may occur with in-pocket insulation breach or unipolar sensing.
Respiratory maneuvers: coughing, straining, sitting up, Valsalva, and deep breathing.	Oversensing of diaphragmatic myopotentials, especially in integrated bipolar leads.

oversensing indicates an intracardiac signal; extracardiac signals produce only noncyclical signals.[24] The simultaneous occurrence of both noncyclical and cyclical oversensing indicates an intracardiac, nonphysiologic source, most commonly LD. Cyclical oversensing related to LD may produce either single or multiple oversensed events for each true ventricular cycle; in contrast, cyclical oversensing of a physiologic signal always results in a single oversensed signal per cardiac cycle.[24]
- Specific sources of oversensing generate signals with different and sometimes diagnostic characteristics related to morphology, frequency content, amplitude, rate, and regularity.[24]

Typical oversensed signals originating in conductors

The typical oversensed signals originating in pace-sense conductor fracture have 6 characteristics. Of these 6 characteristics, the first 3 are almost always present[8] (see **Fig. 5**): (1) they have a high dominant frequency and are intermittent; (2) sequential signals vary in amplitude, frequency, or morphology; (3) they are not recorded on the shock channel in dedicated

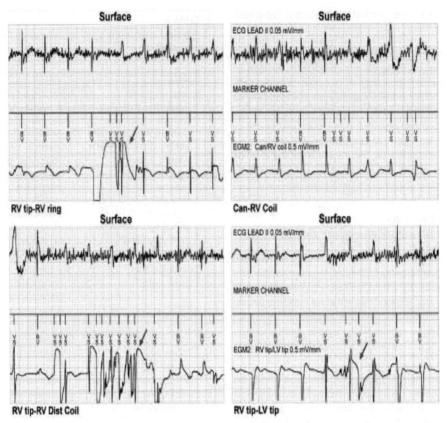

Fig. 3. Role of real-time EGMs, physical maneuver, and differential recording to diagnose the conductor responsible for oversensing. The patient received a shock while shaking his cardiologist's hand the day after a CRT-D implant with a DF-1 defibrillation lead. In each of the 4 panels, the top tracing is the surface electrocardiogram (ECG), which displays motion artifact from hand-shaking during recording to reproduce the malfunction; and the middle tracing is the RV marker channel. The bottom tracing shows the real-time EGM: RV tip to RV ring (dedicated bipolar) top left; RV tip to RV distal coil (integrated bipolar) bottom left; Can to RV coil (shock) top right; RV tip to LV tip bottom right. In each panel there are more "VS" markers than surface QRS complexes, indicating oversensing. "VS" markers apply to short RR intervals (as opposed to "TS" or "FS") because detection is OFF for troubleshooting. Typical ICD system-related oversensing (see **Fig. 5**) is recorded in all of the EGMs (*arrows*) except Can to RV coil (*top right*), the only EGM in which the conductor to the RV tip is not part of the circuit. This indicates a source in the conductor or connection to the RV tip. The time course is too early for a conductor fracture, and an implant-related insulation breach should affect an outer cable, not the inner helical coil. Chest radiograph showed complete insertion of the RV pace-sense pin. At reoperation, there was a loose setscrew to the RV pace-sense port, overlying the tip electrode. (*From* Friedman PA, Swerdlow CD, Hayes DL. Troubleshooting. In: Hayes DL, Friedman PA, editors. Cardiac pacing and defibrillation: a clinical approach. 2nd edition. West Sussex (United Kingdom); with permission.)

bipolar leads; (4) they may be cyclical, noncyclical, or both; (5) at least some intervals are usually nonphysiologic, that is, shorter than typical physiologic intervals (eg, ≤150 ms); and (6) signal amplitude may overshoot the range of the sensing amplifier and hence appear truncated. High-output pacing may precipitate or exacerbate LD-related oversensing.[14] Importantly, IS-1 connection problems between leads and headers may cause indistinguishable, conductor-related oversensing, except that connection problems do not cause cyclical signals (see **Fig. 5**, see later in this article).

Typical oversensed signals caused by insulation breaches

Signal characteristics vary, reflecting the source signal. Intermittent, high-amplitude pectoral myopotentials on the sensing channel suggest an in-pocket, outside-in abrasion for either integrated bipolar or dedicated bipolar leads[25] (**Fig. 6**). Inside-out insulation breaches[26] cause intracardiac, mechanical interactions between lead conductor elements; interactions between 2 pace-sense components (ring cable and central helix), or between pace-sense and shock component,[2,27] and may present as oversensing (**Fig. 7**).

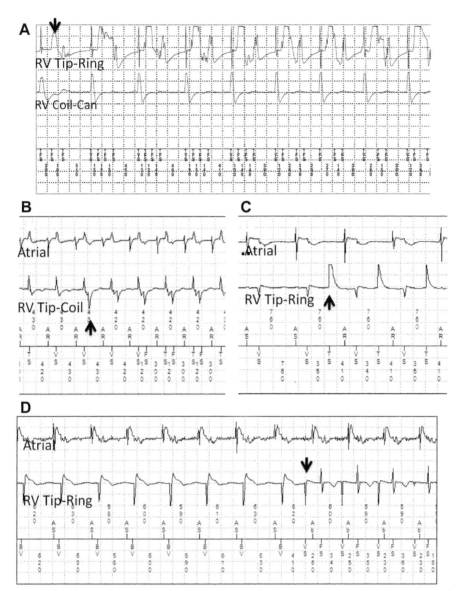

Fig. 4. Spectrum of cyclical oversensing in lead failure. In each panel, arrow denotes first oversensed event. (*A*) Multiphasic signal superimposed on ST segment and T-wave in Fidelis (Medtronic Inc) ring-cable fracture confirmed by returned product analysis. This episode was classified as oversensing by the LNA (Medtronic Inc) and VT/VF therapy was withheld. See **Fig. 16**. (*B*) Cyclical oversensing (*arrow*) coupled to R-wave by nonphysiologic short intervals in integrated bipolar Endotak Reliance G lead (Boston Scientific), simulating R-wave double counting. (*C*) Low-frequency cyclical T-synchronous oversensing in Riata ST Optim lead (Abbott) that subsequently triggered T-wave oversensing algorithm. (*D*) Cyclical spikes in failure of Riata lead (Abbott). (*From* Swerdlow CD, Asirvatham SJ, Ellenbogen KA, et al. Troubleshooting implanted cardioverter defibrillator sensing problems I. Circ Arrhythm Electrophysiol 2014;7(6):1237–61; with permission.)

They often produce EGMs with characteristic spikes on the sensing channel or both sensing and shock channels, thought to represent such mechanical interactions[2,25,28] (**Fig. 8**).

Interpretation of challenging oversensing patterns

Most challenging oversensing patterns fall into 1 of 3 groups (**Tables 3** and **4**):

- Non–LD-related oversensing may have similarities to typical LD-related oversensing (**Table 5**). Examples include atypical electromagnetic interference (EMI) recorded on the sensing dipole from only 1 lead, lead-lead mechanical interactions, or diaphragmatic myopotential (**Fig. 9**).
- LD-related oversensing has similarities to typical non–LD-related oversensing.[24]

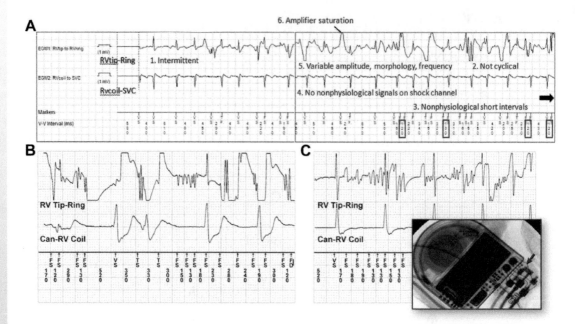

Fig. 5. Characteristics of typical nonphysiologic signals originating in the CIED system. (*A*) Signal characteristics. See text for details. Dedicated bipolar sensing EGM (RVtip to RVring) and a shock channel (RV coil to SVC coil) are displayed with marker channel. (*B*) Connection problem due to incomplete insertion of IS-1 lead pin into header (*arrow* on insert spot radiograph). Signal characteristics do not distinguish fractures from connection problems. Each panel shows sensing channel (RV Tip–Ring), shock channel (CAN-RV Coil) and marker channel. (*C*) Fidelis (Medtronic, Inc) lead fracture. ([*B*] *Adapted from* Swerdlow CD, Sachanandani H, Gunderson BD, et al. Preventing overdiagnosis of implantable cardioverter-defibrillator lead fractures using device diagnostics. J Am Coll Cardiol 2011;57(23):2330–9; with permission.)

Cyclical lead flexing that produces 1 cyclical LD-related, oversensed signal per cardiac cycle may simulate physiologic oversensing (see **Fig. 4**B–D). In-pocket, lead-lead abrasions are an exception to the rule that oversensing on multiple leads is EMI.

- The pattern is not typical of either LD-related or non–LD-related oversensing. The flow chart in **Fig. 10** shows our approach to these patients.

Shock electrograms

EGMs play a lesser role in diagnosing high-voltage component failure than pace-sense component failure because spurious signals isolated to shock EGMs neither cause oversensing nor trigger alerts. EGMs recorded between large, widely spaced electrodes have a wide field of view. Thus, shock EGMs in intact leads commonly record extracardiac signals from the extracardiac electrodes, including pectoral myopotentials indistinguishable from those recorded on sensing conductors as a result of in-pocket insulation breach (see **Fig. 6**). Nevertheless, real-time EGMs displaying abnormal signals originating in an intravascular shock conductor may be the first indicator of LD. If shock-component

LD is suspected, differential EGMs may clarify the signal source. For example, simultaneous recording of shock and integrated bipolar EGMs clarifies if the RV coil conductor or pectoral Can is the signal source. For integrated bipolar leads, the RV coil is the proximal sensing electrode, so LD of the conductor to RV coil presents as oversensing.

Device-Measured Electrical Parameters of Lead Performance

When LD-related oversensing first occurs, the traditional, automated, pace-sense electrical parameters of pacing impedance, pacing threshold, and R-wave amplitude are usually normal. However, abnormal values may confirm the diagnosis of LD when EGMs are not diagnostic.

Pacing impedance and trends

Early-stage conductor fractures may not cause changes in impedance, as the electrode-myocardial interface provides more than 90% of baseline circuit impedance, and conductors contribute less than 10%. Typically, impedance increases only after oversensing occurs.[8,11,16] Most

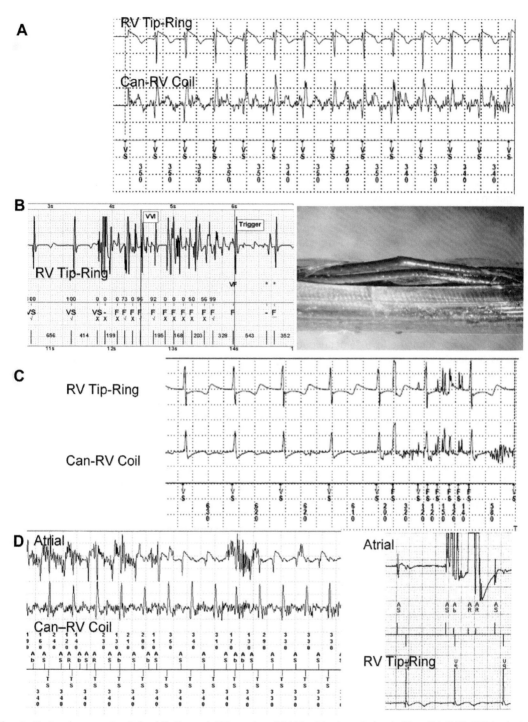

Fig. 6. Pectoral myopotentials. (*A*) Normal RV sensing (RV Tip–Ring) and shock (Can-RV Coil) EGMs during exercise-induced sinus tachycardia. Pectoral myopotentials are visible on the shock channel but not the sensing channel. (*B*). High-amplitude pectoral myopotentials on RV sensing EGM caused by lead-can abrasion (photo of explanted Riata lead). (*C*) Real-time recording during pectoral muscle exercise shows simultaneous pectoral my-opotentials on sensing and shock EGMs of Riata lead, which was capped and abandoned at lead replacement. A lead-can abrasion was visible at surgery. (*D*) Left panel shows stored EGM recorded during sinus tachycardia due to exercise on rowing machine in a patient with a dual-chamber ICD. Atrial EGM, shock EGM, and dual-chamber marker channels are shown. The shock EGM records constant-amplitude myopotentials, a normal finding. Normal ventricular sensing is inferred from the correspondence of the shock EGMs with the ventricular markers in the VT

silicone abrasions of multilumen leads present with pacing impedances within the nominal range,[19,25] but for a different reason: unless the insulation breach causes direct conductor-conductor contact, the impedance of the parallel breach pathway is sufficiently high that circuit impedance remains within the nominal range. Although out-of-range impedance does not provide reliable warning for LD, oversensing accompanied by characteristic impedance abnormalities is highly specific for LD or lead-connection problems. **Fig. 11** summarizes characteristic impedance changes in LD and other conditions.

Impedance increases Conductor fracture: An abrupt 50% to 75% relative change in impedance is more specific for a CIED system problem (conductor fracture or connection problem) than the absolute impedance value and slightly more sensitive[8,17] (see **Fig. 11**; **Fig. 12**).

IS-1 connection problems: Connection problems due to incomplete pace-sense pin insertion into the header constitute up to 10% of suspected fractures for leads with older DF-1/IS-1 connectors[8,17] and usually cannot be distinguished by oversensing pattern. However, a clinical algorithm incorporating impedance trends and the temporal course of oversensing correctly classified all fractures and 87% of connection problems that were misdiagnosed as fractures clinically[8] (**Fig. 13**). The following points apply:

Connection problems usually appear in the first 6 months after connecting the lead to the generator (eg, lead implant, generator change, or lead replacement). LD rarely occurs in the first year after new lead implant, but may occur early after generator change.

- Connection problems rarely cause oversensing without an impedance increase.
- Conversely, LD rarely causes an impedance increase without oversensing.
- Impedance increases may be intermittent in both conditions. A return to baseline impedance for an extended period is common in connection problems, but vanishingly rare in LD[8,16] (see **Fig. 11A**; **Fig. 14**).

- Connection problems due to incomplete lead pin insertion causes oversensing signals limited to the proximal electrode by differential recording.[8] Signals localized to the tip electrode indicate fracture (**Fig. 15**) if a loose set screw (see **Fig. 3**) is excluded.

DF-4 connector An abrupt impedance increase with nominal pacing threshold indicates conductor fracture because incomplete pin insertion affects all 4 pin connections.

Impedance rises at the electrode-myocardial interface: A gradual impedance rise to an out-of-range value usually indicates a problem at the electrode-myocardial interface[8] (see **Fig. 11C, D**), typically caused by calcium deposition as hydroxyapatite. Oversensing does not occur. Intervention is not required as long as sensing and pacing threshold remain acceptable.

Impedance decreases Impedance changes are rare in pace-sense insulation breaches. Although there are no validated criteria of insulation-breach–related changes, in a chronic lead, a visually apparent trend of progressively decreasing impedance or intermittent, low, out-of-range values suggests an insulation breach (see **Figs. 7** and **8**). Impedance decreases in the range of 25% to 50% may occur acutely or subacutely in RV perforations and intracavitary lead dislodgements,[29,30] as well as acutely in in situ leads.

Pacing threshold and R-wave amplitude
Although LD can cause abnormalities in these parameters, to the best of our knowledge, abnormalities do not occur without concomitant impedance changes or typical oversensing patterns. Conductor fractures typically cause loss of capture at maximum output, whereas insulation breaches do not. Similarly, insulation breaches typically cause variable reductions in R-wave amplitude, whereas the open circuits of complete conductor fractures typically show nonphysiologic signals with no reduction in R waves. Occasionally, an insulation breach may be identified when parallel current flow through an intermittent breach causes intermittent abrupt reductions in R-wave

zone (TS). The atrial EGM shows intermittent, high-amplitude pectoral myopotentials, which should not be recorded from an intact closely spaced, intracardiac bipole. Atrial oversensing resulted in inappropriate detection of VT based on a rapid, irregular atrial rate (presumed atrial fibrillation) with a regular dissociated ventricular rhythm. This older ICD does not use ventricular EGM morphology to discriminate VT from SVT. Right panel shows real-time recording during pectoral muscle exercise. High-frequency pectoral myopotentials on atrial channel confirm atrial lead insulation breach due to coil-can abrasion. (*From* Ellenbogen KA, Gunderson BD, Stromberg KD, et al. Performance of lead integrity alert to assist in the clinical diagnosis of implantable cardioverter defibrillator lead failures: analysis of different implantable cardioverter defibrillator leads. Circ Arrhythm Electrophysiol 2013;6(6):1169–77; with permission.)

A Stored EGMs

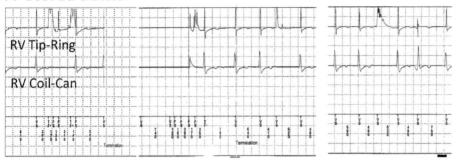

B Real-Time EGMs

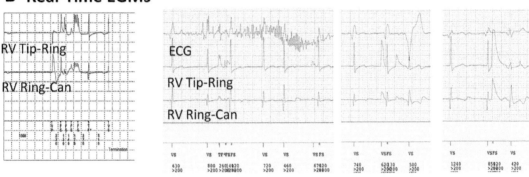

C RV Impedance

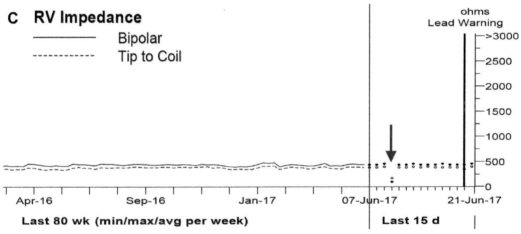

Fig. 7. EGMs and impedance trend from Medtronic LIA resulting from subclavian crush, insulation breach shown in **Fig. 1**. (*A*) Stored EGMs of "nonsustained episodes" that contributed to triggering LIA. The dedicated bipolar sensing EGM (RV Tip–Ring) displays transient, high-frequency signals that saturate the sensing amplifier. Marker channel indicates "nonphysiologic" oversensing with some signals ≤130 ms. The simultaneous shock EGM (RV Coil–Can) does not show abnormal signals. (*B*) Real-time EGMs. Real-time differential EGMs display sensing EGM together with an EGM chosen for diagnostic value, RV Ring-Can. Abnormal signals were recorded with hand pushing up against resistance. These signals occur simultaneously on both channels, indicating that signals enter sensing circuit from conductor to ring electrode. These signals did not occur on the integrated bipolar EGM (not shown) when it was used as a reference. (*C*) Pacing impedance trends for both dedicated bipolar ("Bipolar") and integrated bipolar (Tip to Coil) circuits show single low, out-of-range measurement occurring simultaneously on both circuits. Transient signals, likely myopotentials related to clavicular crush, enter the sensing circuit only from the exposed ring electrode because it is closest to the surface of the lead. However, if an impedance measurement is performed while the lead is compressed, inner ETFE insulation breaches on both conductors permit shorting the 2 conductors, causing a low value on both circuits (*red arrow*).

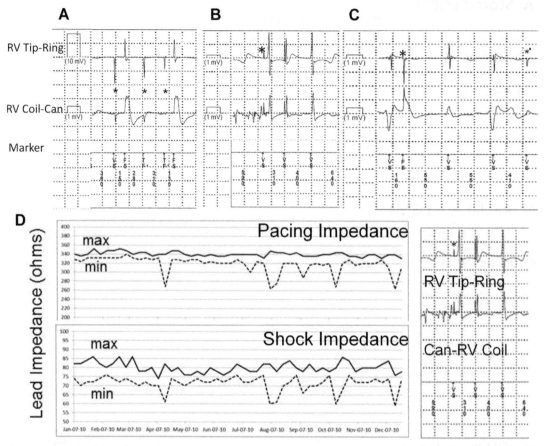

Fig. 8. EGM spikes (*) and impedance trends in insulation breaches. Nonphysiologic, simultaneous spikes on both sensing (RV Tip–Ring) and shock (Can–RV Coil) EGMs in inside-out insulation breaches of Abbott leads (A and B, Riata; C, Durata; D, Riata ST Optim). (D) Also displays pacing and shock impedance trends for the same lead, showing transient, small, simultaneous decreases in both trends. (*From* Ellenbogen KA, Gunderson BD, Stromberg KD, et al. Performance of lead integrity alert to assist in the clinical diagnosis of implantable cardioverter defibrillator lead failures: analysis of different implantable cardioverter defibrillator leads. Circ Arrhythm Electrophysiol 2013;6(6):1169–77; with permission.)

amplitude. In the evaluation of elevated pacing impedance, a moderate increase in pacing threshold and moderate reduction in R-wave amplitude favors an electrode-myocardial interface issue over LD. Atypical LD oversensing patterns usually are associated with normal pacing threshold and R-wave amplitude.

Shock impedance and trends

Shock impedance is the primary diagnostic tool for high-voltage conductors. In Sprint Fidelis leads connected to Medtronic ICDs (Medtronic, Inc, Minneapolis, MN), either RV coil, impedance greater than 100 Ω or an increase in impedance by 75% over baseline are diagnostic of a high-voltage conductor fracture.[9] Low-voltage measurements of shock impedance are insensitive for insulation breaches unless direct contact with another conductor is present. Ipsilateral

pleural effusion can lower shock impedance, and pneumothorax can raise it. Abnormally low impedance also can be caused by reversal of the SVC and RV coils in the header for older DF-1 leads.[31] Manufacturers have remote monitoring alerts for out-of-range shock impedance. To reduce false positives, the alert for the SVC coil should be disabled for single-coil leads.

ADVANCED IMPLANTABLE CARDIOVERTER-DEFIBRILLATOR FEATURES TO DETECT AND MITIGATE LEAD DYSFUNCTION

In addition to traditional measures of lead performance, some ICDs have specific software to detect and mitigate the consequences of LD. Most such features are triggered by metrics of oversensing and/or abrupt changes in pacing impedance. Because each feature has false positives and false negatives, the diagnosis of LD

Table 3
Rapid oversensing with normal pacing impedance: signal source within implantable cardioverter-defibrillator system (lead dysfunction or other system element)

Condition	Features of Oversensed Signal	Time After Lead Implant	Other Clues
Conductor fracture	Specific signal characteristics[a] (see **Fig. 5**)	Late	Postpacing oversensing.
Insulation breach (in-pocket, outside-in)	Pectoral myopotentials (uniformly high-frequency, variable amplitude) on dedicated bipolar electrogram (EGM) (see **Fig. 6**)	Late	Pectoral muscle exercise reproduces oversensing. Pocket manipulation may cause oversensing.
Insulation breach (intravascular, inside-out)	Spikes. Signals may be both rapid and isolated (see **Fig. 8**)	Usually late	Simultaneous spikes on multiple EGM channels.
IS-I connection problems	Indistinguishable from conductor fracture (see **Fig. 5**)	Usually early after new lead, or generator change	Never cyclical. Differential EGM recording isolates source to proximal electrode. Impedance usually abnormal within days. Radiography often confirms diagnosis. May be reproduced by pocket manipulation.
Loose set screw	No systematic reports of signal characteristics; some cases have transient, noncyclical, high-frequency signals (see **Fig. 3**)	Early	If 1 set screw, source is tip electrode. If 2 set screws, source may be either proximal or distal electrode.
Air trapped in header	Uniform, medium-frequency signals[24]	Early	Rare after 30 d.

[a] See text.

should be based on analysis of the previously described source data rather than the presence or absence of a lead alert.

Counts of Nonphysiologic Short Intervals

Count of nonphysiologic short intervals
Extremely short R-R intervals near the ventricular blanking period are referred to as "nonphysiologic" because they do not represent successive cardiac depolarizations, except during VF. Medtronic ICDs count intervals within 20 ms of the blanking period (nominally ≤130 ms) in the Sensing Integrity Count. A rapidly increasing Sensing Integrity Count (>10 per day for 3 consecutive days) is a sensitive, but nonspecific indicator of pace-sense conductor fracture.[17] Other manufacturers provide histograms of R-R intervals. Nonphysiologic short

intervals increment the count in the highest rate bin. This finding is also nonspecific, but many counts in the fastest bin with no counts in adjacent bins suggests nonphysiologic oversensing.

Alerts Incorporating Impedance Changes and Indirect Evidence of Oversensing

These algorithms are based on evidence that monitoring both indirect evidence of rapid oversensing and impedance trends provided earlier warning of LD than a fixed impedance threshold.[17]

Lead integrity alert
This first lead-alert algorithm to incorporate oversensing includes 1 criterion related to abrupt changes in pace-sense impedance and 2 related to transient, rapid oversensing[16]

Table 4
Rapid oversensing with normal pacing impedance: signal source external to the implantable cardioverter-defibrillator system

Condition	Features of Oversensed Signal	Time After Lead Implant	Other Clues
Electromagnetic interference	Reflects characteristics of source. Usually high frequency.	Any	Usually identified on multiple channels and leads. In dedicated bipolar leads, amplitude usually greater on shock channel than sensing channel.[24] History may suggest source. May occur only when patient is in a specific environment (eg, shower, workshop).
Diaphragmatic myopotentials	Uniformly low-amplitude (see **Fig. 9**, vs pectoral myopotentials, which vary in amplitude). Relatively uniform morphology (vs conductor signals, which vary in morphology, amplitude, or both).	Any	Usually with integrated bipolar leads at right ventricular apex. Reproduced by respiratory maneuvers. Not reproduced by pectoral muscle maneuvers or pocket manipulation. Usually in paced rhythm or bradycardia.
P/T-wave oversensing or R-wave double counting	Cyclical, single oversensed signal in each cardiac cycle. Frequency content corresponds to intracardiac signal, but appearance may be altered by high-pass filtering if only filtered electrogram (EGM) is recorded.[24]	Any	Timing consistent with physiologic source.
Ventricular fibrillation	Variable.	Any	Present on both shock and sensing channels. Usually stops after shock.
Lead-lead mechanical interactions	Spikes on both leads.	Late	Presence of other leads. Cinefluoroscopy with real-time EGM recordings confirms diagnosis.

(**Fig. 16**A). It alerts if any 2 criteria are fulfilled. The false-positive rate is low, and lower for dedicated bipolar than integrated bipolar leads (<1/400 vs 1/80 patient-years), mostly due to more triggering by EMI in integrated bipolar leads.[8,17,32] Extensive clinical data documents that lead integrity alert (LIA) improves early detection of Fidelis lead fractures compared with monitoring impedance alone.[16,17,33] LIA also identifies both conductor fracture and insulation breaches in other leads from various manufacturers.[8,25,34]

Latitude lead check
Like LIA, this alert is triggered by either evidence of oversensing or impedance changes. Oversensing ("noise") is detected if a device-stored sustained episode includes 4 ventricular sensed beats with cycle length ≤160 ms. An oversensing alert is triggered by 1 episode treated with antitachycardia pacing, 1 episode with a diverted shock, or no-therapy sustained episodes on 2 of the past 30 days. An impedance alert is triggered by a daily out-of-range (200–2000 Ω) pace-sense impedance, a daily out-of-range (20–125 Ω) shock

Table 5
Characteristics of typical oversensed electrogram signal patterns of lead dysfunction and potentially confounding patterns that may not be related to lead dysfunction

Signal Characteristic	Patterns Related to Lead Dysfunction	Patterns Not Related to Lead Dysfunction
High-frequency	Characteristic, nonphysiologic signals in conductor fractures or IS-1 connection problems, limited to sensing channel of dedicated bipolar leads (see **Fig. 5**)	Characteristic 50/60-Hz electromagnetic interference on multiple channels, multiple leads.[24]
Myopotentials	Myopotentials on dedicated bipolar leads indicating outside-in, in-pocket insulation breach (see **Fig. 6**)	Diaphragmatic myopotentials on integrated bipolar leads. Pectoral myopotentials on shock channel or unipolar sensing channel (see **Fig. 4A**).
Single oversensed signal per cardiac cycle	Cyclical or noncyclical spikes with inside-out, insulation breaches, sometimes on both sensing and shock channels from same lead (see **Fig. 4**)	Cyclical physiologic signals: P/T-wave oversensing or R-wave double counting.[24] Cyclical or noncyclical spikes caused by mechanical interactions between leads. Requires presence of multiple leads[24] (see **Fig. 9B**).

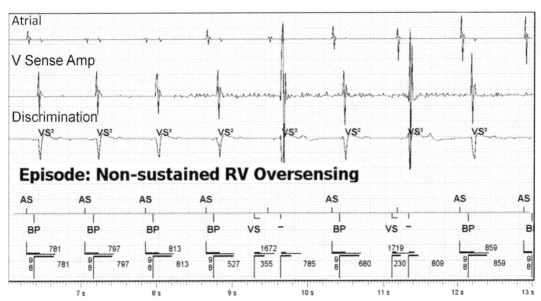

Fig. 9. Diaphragmatic myopotentials on dedicated bipolar lead after upgrade to CRT-D from older dual-chamber ICD, activating Abbott SecureSense lead-noise algorithm. Atrial EGM, filtered dedicated bipolar sensing EGM (V Sense Amp), shock EGM (Discrimination), and marker channel are shown. The sensing EGM shows relatively uniform, low-amplitude, high-frequency, signals. VS markers on sensing channel that do not correspond to VS2 markers on shock channel denote oversensed events. Recording non-cardiac signals on an in-situ lead immediately post-operatively after an upgrade procedure raises the questions of intraoperative lead injury and connection issue. Recording of diaphragmatic myopotentials is extremely rare with dedicated bipolar sensing. The primary cause of oversensing with the new CRT generator but not the previous ICD generator on the same lead is that the new generator includes a Low Frequency Attenuation Filter, which selectively amplifies high-frequency signals and is nominally ON. Differences in bandpass filters may cause clinically-significant differences in sensing when different generators are connected to the same RV, dedicated-bipolar lead.[49]

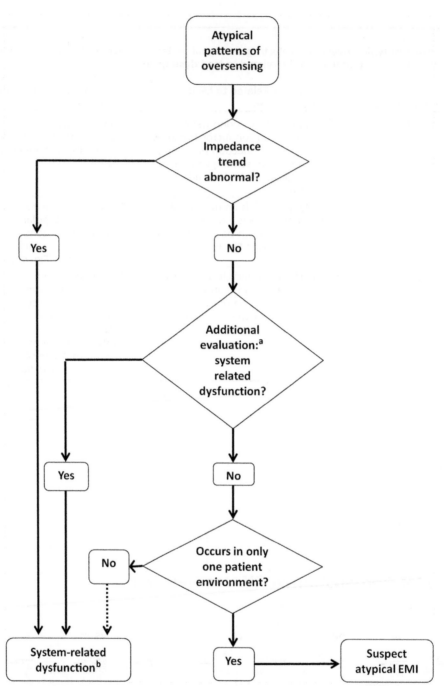

Fig. 10. Deductive approach to the evaluation of atypical patterns of oversensing. Dotted line indicates diagnosis of exclusion, with some uncertainty. [a] Additional evaluation: Real-time EGMs with physical maneuvers (see **Table 2**), Differential EGMs, Pacing and sensing thresholds, Shock impedance, Imaging. [b] See **Fig. 13** for differentiation of LD from IS-1 connection problem.

impedance, or abrupt, in-range changes in pacing impedance on 3 of 7 days. Unlike LIA, latitude lead check is implemented in remote monitoring rather than the generator, so there is no patient alert and alerts are active only while patients are in range of remote monitoring. Clinical performance has not been reported.

Algorithms that Compare Sensing and Shock Electrograms

Two algorithms use the shock EGM as a check on the sensing EGM to monitor direct evidence of oversensing, and withhold therapies if oversensing is detected. Oversensing is diagnosed by the

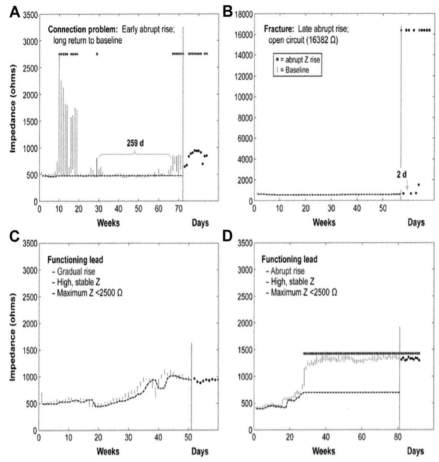

Fig. 11. Pace-sense impedance trends. To the left of the longest vertical line, data are displayed as vertical lines connecting weekly maximum and minimum values. To right, points indicate daily values. Red stars denote impedance measurements that fulfill criteria for an abrupt rise. (*A*) Connection problem with first abrupt rise occurring 10 weeks postimplantation with long return to baseline (259 days). (*B*) Fracture with abrupt impedance rise to open circuit. Longest return to baseline is 2 days. (*C*) Gradual impedance rise in functioning lead. (*D*) Abrupt rise to high, stable impedance in functioning lead. Trends in (*C*) and (*D*) occur due to changes at the electrode-myocardial interface. (*From* Swerdlow CD, Sachanandani H, Gunderson BD, et al. Preventing overdiagnosis of implantable cardioverter-defibrillator lead fractures using device diagnostics. J Am Coll Cardiol 2011;57:2330–9; with permission.)

presence of more signals on the sensing channel than on the shock channel. Both algorithms may trigger alerts for conditions other than lead failure. Such false positives are desirable if they are triggered by clinically significant oversensing events that, if unrecognized, might result in inappropriate shocks (eg, T-wave oversensing). For both algorithms, the most serious potential risk is that undersensing VF on the shock channel could result in false-positive diagnosis of oversensing and failure to deliver life-saving therapy. With integrated bipolar sensing, neither algorithm is triggered reliably by oversensing related to the RV coil conductor, because this coil is common to both the sensing and shock channels. The algorithms operate and perform differently.

Lead noise algorithm

The lead noise algorithm (LNA; Medtronic Inc) (**Fig. 16**B) analyzes a shock channel temporal window centered on a sense-channel event rather than "sensing" the shock channel continuously. In clinical testing, the maximum delay for detecting induced VF was 2 seconds.[35] In the PainFree SST trial, there were no instances of LNA withholding appropriate VT/VF detection and no false positives among adjudicated episodes. However, the performance of the LNA was disappointing. Although only 23 of 824 device-detected "lead noise" episodes received a shock, 8 (73%) of 11 patients with LD had at least 1 shock. The main causes of inappropriate shocks were shock EGMs

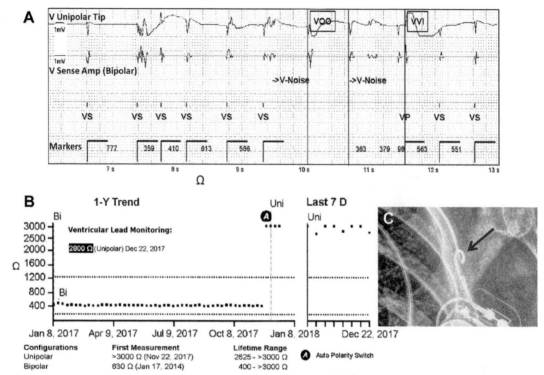

Fig. 12. Conductor fracture due to a ventricular lead knot with oversensing of nonphysiologic signals and operation of noise-reversion algorithm in an Abbott Accent single-chamber pacemaker. (*A*) Stored EGMs from the pacemaker shows unipolar EGM (V Unipolar tip) and filtered dedicated bipolar sensing EGM (V Sense Amp). The noise-reversion algorithm detects multiple fast signals within a specified time frame (62.5-ms sampling windows after sensed events) as noise and enters into a noise-reversion mode, asynchronous pacing at the base rate or sensor indicated rate. (*B*) Pacing impedance trends show initial bipolar (tip to ring) stable impedance measurements for 1 year with autopolarity switch to unipolar (tip to Can) pacing mode on November 22, 2017. Abrupt increase to out-of-range unipolar impedance in chronic lead without surgical intervention indicates fracture of conductor to tip electrode. (*C*) Section of chest radiograph with magnified view of the proximal part of the failed ventricular lead (Abbott Tendril 2088TC), showing a knot in the lead (*red arrow*), suggesting the site of conductor fracture. (*Courtesy of* Abbott, Inc, St Paul, MN.)

without a low-amplitude baseline or a low-amplitude true ventricular EGM on the shock channel.

SecureSense Right Ventricular Lead Noise Discrimination Algorithm

SecureSense (Abbott Medical, St Paul, MN) uses 2 independent sensing amplifiers, one on the sensing channel and one on a far-field Discrimination channel (nominally RV coil–CAN). See **Fig. 17** for details. Sensing channel events with intervals shorter than the slowest VT/VF interval are classified as oversensing if they do not correlate with "fast" intervals on the shock ("Discrimination") channel. When rate and duration criteria for detection of VT/VF are met, the algorithm withholds therapy if too many events are classified as oversensing. SecureSense also functions as a diagnostic that triggers lead alerts when a sufficient number of intervals are classified as oversensing ("nonsustained

oversensing"). Multiple desirable and undesirable causes of false-positive alerts have been identified.[36] In clinical practice, SecureSense combined with remote monitoring withheld therapy from all 10 inappropriate detections of VF due to lead failure and did not withhold therapy from any of 321 sustained VT/VF episodes, but 12% of patients had at least 1 alert.[18] Despite safeguards, false-positive withholding of a shock from VF has been reported.[37]

Shock Vector Switching for Shock-Conductor Insulation Breach

An automatic shocking vector adjustment algorithm (Dynamic Tx; Abbott Medical) can prevent pulse generator damage and ensure shock delivery in at least some high-voltage insulation breaches that cause shorting in the shock output circuit of dual-coil leads. During a shock, if a short is present in 1 of the 2 dual-coil shock pathways

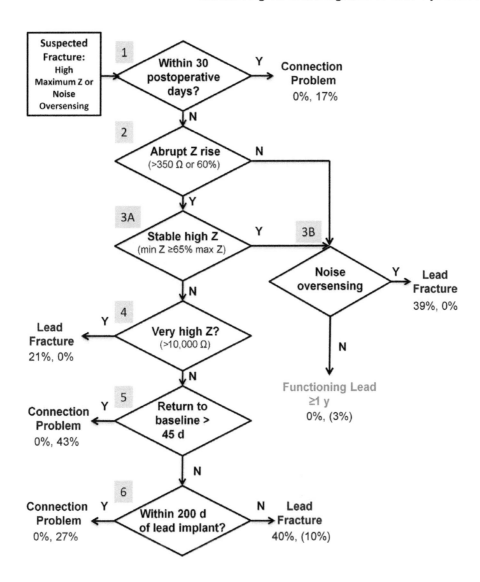

% of 70 Lead Fractures, % of 30 Connection Problems

Fig. 13. Clinical algorithm for discrimination of pace-sense lead fractures from connection problems and functioning leads with impedance rises at electrode-myocardial interface. Numbers in gray boxes denote algorithm steps. Percentages at each step indicate algorithm's classification for 70 fractures (*maroon text*) and 30 connection problems (*blue text*). Values in parentheses denote incorrect classification. The algorithm correctly classified all 4 impedance trends shown in **Fig. 11.** max, maximum; min, minimum. (*From* Swerdlow CD, Sachanandani H, Gunderson BD, et al. Preventing overdiagnosis of implantable cardioverter-defibrillator lead fractures using device diagnostics. J Am Coll Cardiol 2011;57:2330–9; with permission.)

(RV coil–Can, RV coil–SVC coil), this feature aborts the shocks and delivers the next shock through the alternate and presumably intact pathway.[38,39]

LEAD DYSFUNCTION IN PACING LEADS
Atrial and Right Ventricular Leads

Because older pacemakers had minimal EGM storage, LD typically presented with oversensing-induced inhibition of pacing, failure to capture or

sense, or impedance abnormalities. Modern pacemakers store EGMs when noise rejection algorithms are activated and communicate wirelessly with remote monitoring networks, improving early diagnosis. See **Fig. 12** for an example. As in ICDs without oversensing alerts, the diagnosis of LD is often made by evaluation of EGMs stored for other reasons. Atrial LD is often identified by review of atrial "high-rate" episodes mislabeled as "atrial fibrillation."

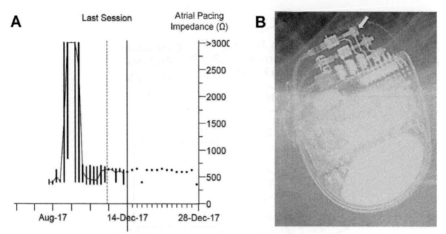

Fig. 14. Atrial lead-connection problem. (*A*) Atrial pace-sense impedance trend for CRT-P after generator change on July 18, 2017. No intervention was performed. To the left of the longest vertical line, data are displayed as vertical lines connecting weekly maximum and minimum values. To right, black points indicate daily values. Impedance was approximately 400 Ω for the first 3 weeks, then rises abruptly to above the maximum measured value of 3000 Ω. After 6 weeks, it returns to a new baseline of approximately 700 Ω. No intervention was performed. Oversensing did not occur; P-wave amplitude did not change; and pacing threshold increased from 0.5 V to 1.0 V at new, stable plateau. (*B*) Radiograph of generator shows incomplete insertion of atrial pin into header (*arrow*).

The presentation of LD may be influenced by unipolar sensing and pacing, which is not available in ICDs. Many pacemakers respond to a marked pacing threshold increase or impedance change by reverting from bipolar to unipolar modes. As noted previously, pectoral myopotentials are a normal finding on unipolar EGMs.

Recent reports document oversensing of the signal for the minute ventilation (MV) sensor used to adjust rate-responsive pacing in Boston Scientific

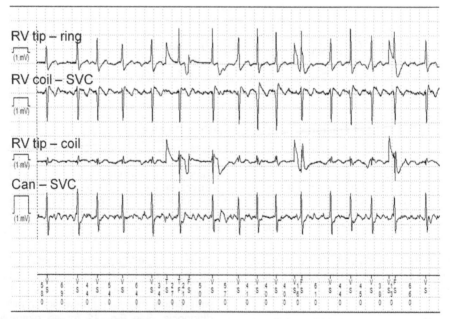

Fig. 15. Real-time, differential EGM. Channels are shown in order: dedicated bipolar EGM, shock EGM, integrated bipolar EGM, "leadless ECG," and marker channel. Sensing channel shows noncyclical, high-frequency, highly variable, oversensed signals. These signals occur on integrated bipolar channel but not shock channel, indicating that they originate in central helical conductor to the tip electrode. Abrupt onset of oversensing with normal impedance more than 3 years after generator change excludes connection problem. Box on marker channel denotes nonphysiologic short interval. Abbreviations as in **Fig. 5**. This patient's stored EGMs are shown in **Figs. 5**A and **16B**.

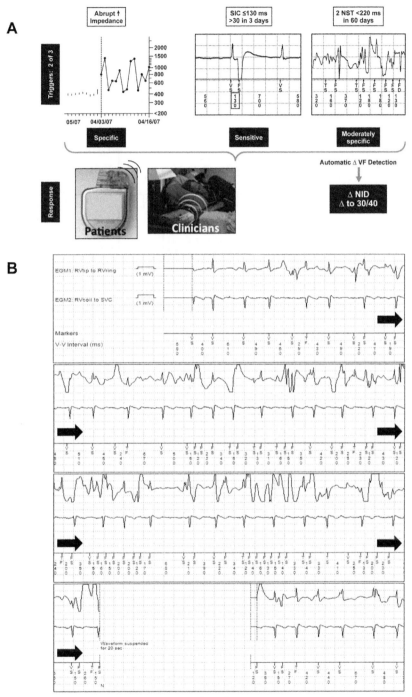

Fig. 16. LIA and LNA, Medtronic Inc (*A*). LIA. *Courtesy* of Medtronic, Inc., Minneapolis, MN. © Medtronic 2018. The relative, abrupt impedance-increase criterion is met if any impedance is ≥75% or less than 50% of an updated baseline value. The 2 oversensing criteria comprise the Sensing Integrity Count (≥10 for 3 consecutive days) and evidence of transient, rapid, repetitive oversensing based "nonsustained tachycardia" (NST) ≥5 device-detected intervals with mean cycle length <220 ms. NID, number of intervals to detect VF; SIC, sensing integrity count. (*B*). LNA withholds shock from conductor fracture. The first 2 of 4 panels were shown previously in **Fig. 5**A (side by side). (*Black arrows*) denote continuous recording. Ventricular fibrillation is detected at left of bottom panel, but, LNA withholds shock ("N" on marker channel) because multiple sensed events do not correspond to valid EGMs on the shock channel. ([*A*] *From* Swerdlow CD, Ellenbogen KA. Implantable cardioverter-defibrillator leads: design, diagnostics, and management. Circulation 2013;128(18):2062–71, 2061–9; with permission; and *Courtesy of* Medtronic, Inc, Minneapolis, MN.)

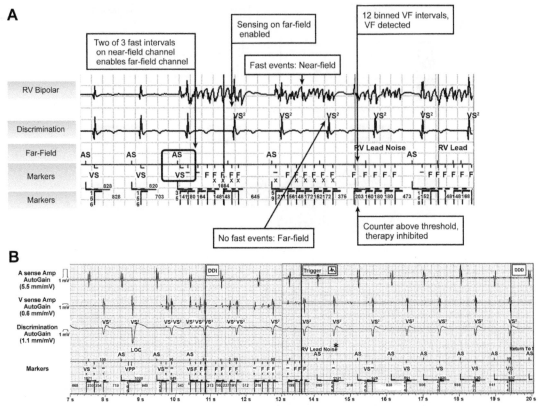

Fig. 17. SecureSense RV Lead Noise Discrimination Algorithm (Abbott). (*A*) Simulation illustrates algorithm operation. SecureSense uses a counter to compare sensed events on the RV dedicated bipolar, sensing channel ("Near-Field [Sensing]") with events sensed independently on a Far-Field ("Discrimination") channel (nominally RV coil–CAN). When 2 of 3 sensing channel intervals in a moving window are shorter than the slowest VT/VF detection interval, the Discrimination channel sense amplifier is enabled, the algorithm is activated, and each sensed event on the Discrimination channel is indicated by the VS2 marker displayed directly on the channel's EGM. An interval on the Discrimination channel is classified as fast if it is within 50 ms of the slowest VT/VF detection interval (30 ms in the original implementation). The algorithm's counter increments by 1 for every VT/VF interval on the sensing channel and resets to 0 after 2 consecutive fast intervals on the Discrimination channel. When detection criteria for VT/VF are met, the algorithm withholds therapy if the count is ≥10. In this example, the programmed number of intervals for detection of VF is 12. Additionally, when the count reaches 10 (5 in the original implementation), SecureSense stores an EGM as "Nonsustained Oversensing" ("Nonsustained Lead Noise" in the original implementation, see **Fig. 5**), whether or not VT/VF has been detected. After a shock, SecureSense is disabled until the device-defined episode ends. (*B*) Clinical example of Riata (St. Jude Medical) lead failure. Panel shows atrial EGM, filtered RV sensing EGM ("V Sense Amp"), shock EGM (Can-RV Coil, "Discrimination"), and marker channel that annotates events sensed on RV sensing channel ("F" denotes intervals in VF zone). Visually, oversensed, spikey nonphysiologic signals on sensing channel correspond with lower-amplitude nonphysiologic signals on Discrimination channel, some of which are not sensed. The disparate appearances of nonphysiologic signals on the 2 channels may be caused by differences in filtering. When the number of intervals to detect VF (12) is reached, the algorithm classifies the episode as oversensing, and withholds capacitor charging (RV Lead Noise, *asterisk*). VPP indicates loss of capture with output 0.25 V above threshold followed by higher-voltage, back-up pulse.

(Marlborough, MA) pacemakers.[40] This constant-current signal is emitted continuously between the ring electrode (atrial ring in dual-chamber pacemakers, ventricular ring in single-chamber pacemakers) and Can. If the measured impedance in this circuit increases, signal voltage is increased to maintain a constant current. This increased applied voltage may exceed the limits of common-mode rejection[41] on the inputs to the atrial and/or ventricular sensing channel, resulting in oversensing of characteristic, constant-amplitude, 20-Hz signals[40] and inhibition of pacing. The increase in impedance may be caused by fracture of the conductor to ring electrode or incomplete lead pin insertion into the header; but in most cases both the lead and connection are intact, and the cause of the measured abnormal impedance is uncertain. Oversensing is corrected by programming the MV sensor off.

Left-Ventricular Leads

Because left-ventricular (LV) leads are not used for primary sensing, LD may present with worsening heart failure from loss of capture. Inside-out insulation breaches leading to cable externalization have been reported in Abbott (St. Jude) silicone-insulated QuickSite (bipolar) and QuickFlex (quadripolar) leads[42,43]; but only isolated cases of electrical dysfunction have been reported. In quadripolar leads, reprogramming the pacing vector may reestablish LV capture if LD does not involve all conductors.

ADDITIONAL CONSIDERATIONS
Remote Monitoring in Detecting and Monitoring Lead Dysfunction

Remote monitoring plays a central role in early detection of asymptomatic electrical LD before clinical consequences occur.[44] For example, remote monitoring shortens the clinical response time to Medtronic LIAs, reducing inappropriate therapies.[22,45] However, remote monitoring of LD involves more than prompt responses to lead alerts. Welte and colleagues[18] reported a systematic approach that minimizes LD-induced inappropriate shocks, even in ICDs without oversensing alerts. They emphasize 3 points.

- *Programming alerts in the remote monitoring network.* Remote monitoring alerts for VT/VF should be set to their most sensitive level; alerts for SVT should be programmed when available.
- *Review all transmitted EGMs*, including EGMs from nonsustained episodes and aborted shocks, supraventricular tachycardia episodes, and real-time recordings. Real-time EGMs also may identify markers of LD that do not trigger inappropriate arrhythmia detection or alerts, such as isolated abnormal signals in inside-out insulation breaches (**Fig. 18**). In ICDs without oversensing alerts, most diagnoses of LD were made by analysis of inappropriate device detections that did not result in therapy or incidental observations on real-time EGMs.
- *Minimize interruptions in remote monitoring and delays in responding to transmissions.* The time between the first evidence of LD and inappropriate shocks is often short. Thus patient-related interruptions (eg, unmonitored travel) should be limited,

and weekend surveillance should be considered.

Imaging in the Diagnosis of Lead Dysfunction

Imaging is unrevealing in most of the cases of suspected pace-sense LD. The chest radiograph is important primarily for excluding alternative causes of oversensing, especially functional LD, such as lead dislodgment or perforation, abandoned leads that may cause lead-lead interactions, or incomplete insertion of IS-1 and DF-1 pins into the header (see **Figs. 5B** and **14**). The chest radiograph should be inspected for lead conductor discontinuity, kinks (see **Fig. 12**) or sharp bends (especially at lateral axillary venous insertions), or twisting suggesting "twiddler's syndrome." Cinefluoroscopy in multiple views is useful for detecting lead-lead interactions. It is the primary method for identifying Riata and other leads with inside-out insulation breaches in which cables protrude outside the outer insulation, especially in the right atrium near the tricuspid valve.[23] However, there is only a weak correlation between externalized cables and oversensing.[5,46–48]

Monitoring and Programming for Lead Dysfunction

Usually, lead replacement is indicated once LD is confirmed. Nevertheless, monitoring is indicated in several clinical scenarios.

At-risk, recalled leads with normal electrical function

Tens of thousands of Medtronic Sprint Fidelis and Abbott (St. Jude) Riata recalled leads continue to function in patients. Consensus recommendations for monitoring these leads and programming connected ICDs[1] facilitate early diagnosis. They are summarized in **Table 6**. Recommendations for Fidelis mitigate the adverse consequences of fracture to ring electrode. Recommendations for Riata mitigate adverse consequences of inside-out insulation breach. These recommendations may be applied in any lead with suspected LD.

Suspected lead dysfunction

If the diagnosis of LD remains uncertain after comprehensive analysis of EGMs and device-measures of lead performance, intensified follow-up usually is appropriate. If possible, the EGM channels should be selected to facilitate diagnosis. If the presentation is oversensing on a dedicated bipolar lead, reprogramming to unipolar sensing (pacemakers) or integrated bipolar sensing (Medtronic ICDs) may be indicated.

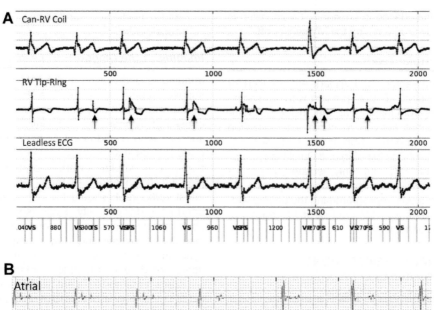

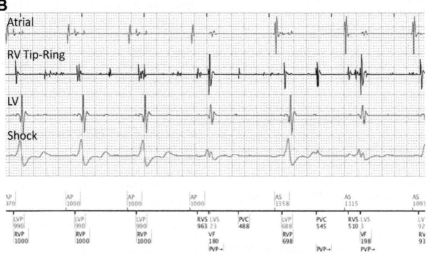

Fig. 18. Value of remote monitoring real-time EGMs for diagnosis of LD. (*A*) Abbott Durata lead. EGMs in order are shock (Can-RV Coil), dedicated bipolar sensing (RV Tip–Ring), and Leadless ECG (Can-SVC). RV sensing EGM shows isolated spikes typical of inside-out insulation breach. (*B*) Biotronik Linox S65 lead. EGMs are labeled in order. The dedicated bipolar sensing channel shows intermittent, high-frequency, highly variable signals, inhibiting CRT after the fourth and sixth atrial complexes. Additional evaluation documented both cyclical and noncyclical, transient high-frequency signals as well as pacing impedance fluctuating between the baseline value of 500 Ω and 240 Ω. These findings are suggestive of inside-out, insulation breach to the ring-electrode cable. ([*B*] *Courtesy of* Dr Sylvain Ploux, Bordeaux, France; with permission.)

Confirmed lead dysfunction, but risk of lead replacement exceeds benefit

Repeat CIED operations have a significant risk of infection and other complications.[1] In some scenarios, it is important to consider monitoring the malfunctioning lead, either until generator change or indefinitely, as an alternative to immediate lead replacement. The clinician should consider the following:

- The immediate risk LD poses to the patient
- The risk of lead replacement now and in the future in the context of patient-specific comorbidities

- The likely rate of progression of LD to other lead elements or other leads and their likely clinical consequences
- The degree to which risk can be mitigated by CIED programming and remote monitoring, possibly combined with intensified in-person follow-up

The third and fourth points are important because expeditious lead replacement may be indicated even if the immediate risk to the patient is low. Consider 2 scenarios of insulation breaches in an elderly patient with a dual-chamber pacemaker, complete heart block, and multiple

Table 6
Recommendations for managing functioning, recalled leads (Medtronic Fidelis and Abbott Riata)

Common recommendations for both leads

Enroll patient in remote monitoring

Turn on all the lead-alert algorithms

Prolong duration of ventricular fibrillation detection to 30–40 beats

Specific recommendations

Fidelis	Riata
Device programming: recommendations for common device/lead parameters	
Lead integrity alert (LIA): ON	Secure Sense Lead Noise Algorithm: ON
High-voltage lead impedance alert: ON >100 Ω	High-voltage lead impedance alert: stable range ±25 Ω
Pacing impedance alert: 75% >baseline	Pacing impedance alert range: 200–1000 Ω
Device programming: other manufacturer-specific recommendations	
Program to integrated bipolar sensing (Medtronic implantable cardioverter-defibrillator)	Right ventricular (RV) autocapture: ON/Monitor Program an electrogram channel to record RV coil–superior vena cava (SVC) coil Exclude SVC coil from defibrillation pathway Shocking Vector Switch algorithm: ON
At generator change	
If lead function is normal and no evidence of fracture, the lead may be reused	Examine of the lead and perform cinefluoroscopy to identify insulation breach Deliver high-voltage synchronized shock to check high-voltage system integrity Implant generator with automatic vector switch capability If lead is functional and electrically intact with lead externalization, no replacement is necessary

comorbidities. If the insulation breach is caused by subclavian crush, programming unipolar pacing and sensing will ensure consistent pacing in the immediate future; yet, the lead remains at risk for continued crush affecting the inner coil to the distal conductor, with unpredictable and abrupt failure to pace. Thus, lead replacement is indicated. Alternatively, consider an insulation breach caused by metal-ion oxidation of inner polyurethane insulation.[12] In this case, programming unipolar pacing and sensing will permit indefinite lead function. The decision to replace can be deferred until generator change is required.

REFERENCES

1. Kusumoto FM, Schoenfeld MH, Wilkoff BL, et al. HRS expert consensus statement on cardiovascular implantable electronic device lead management and extraction. Heart Rhythm 2017;14(12):e503–51.
2. Swerdlow CD, Ellenbogen KA. Implantable cardioverter-defibrillator leads: design, diagnostics, and management. Circulation 2013;128(18):2062–71.
3. Lau EW. Analysis of pacing and defibrillation lead malfunction. Card Electrophysiol Clin 2014;6(2):307–26.
4. Cheung JW, Al-Kazaz M, Thomas G, et al. Mechanisms, predictors, and trends of electrical failure of Riata leads. Heart Rhythm 2013;10(10):1453–9.
5. Schmutz M, Delacretaz E, Schwick N, et al. Prevalence of asymptomatic and electrically undetectable intracardiac inside-out abrasion in silicon-coated Riata(R) and Riata(R) ST implantable cardioverter-defibrillator leads. Int J Cardiol 2013;167(1):254–7.
6. Morales JL, Nava S, Márquez MF, et al. Idiopathic lead migration: concept and variants of an uncommon cause of cardiac implantable electronic device dysfunction. JACC Clin Electrophysiol 2017;3(11):1321–9.
7. Fuertes B, Toquero J, Arroyo-Espliguero R, et al. Pacemaker lead displacement: mechanisms and management. Indian Pacing Electrophysiol J 2003;3(4):231–8.
8. Swerdlow CD, Sachanandani H, Gunderson BD, et al. Preventing overdiagnosis of implantable cardioverter-defibrillator lead fractures using device diagnostics. J Am Coll Cardiol 2011;57(23):2330–9.
9. Koneru JN, Gunderson BD, Sachanandani H, et al. Diagnosis of high-voltage conductor fractures in sprint fidelis leads. Heart Rhythm 2013;10(6):813–8.
10. Magney JE, Flynn DM, Parsons JA, et al. Anatomical mechanisms explaining damage to pacemaker leads, defibrillator leads, and failure of central venous catheters adjacent to the sternoclavicular joint. Pacing Clin Electrophysiol 1993;16(3 Pt 1):445–57.

11. Swerdlow CD, Kalahasty G, Ellenbogen KA. Implantable cardiac defibrillator lead failure and management. J Am Coll Cardiol 2016;67(11): 1358–68.

12. Stokes K, Urbanski P, Upton J. The in vivo auto-oxidation of polyether polyurethane by metal ions. J Biomater Sci Polym Ed 1990;1(3):207–30.

13. Gunderson BD, Gillberg JM, Wood MA, et al. Development and testing of an algorithm to detect implantable cardioverter-defibrillator lead failure. Heart Rhythm 2006;3(2):155–62.

14. Chung EH, Casavant D, John RM. Analysis of pacing/defibrillator lead failure using device diagnostics and pacing maneuvers. Pacing Clin Electrophysiol 2009;32(4):547–9.

15. Kleemann T, Becker T, Doenges K, et al. Annual rate of transvenous defibrillation lead defects in implantable cardioverter-defibrillators over a period of >10 years. Circulation 2007;115(19): 2474–80.

16. Swerdlow CD, Gunderson BD, Ousdigian KT, et al. Downloadable software algorithm reduces inappropriate shocks caused by implantable cardioverter-defibrillator lead fractures: a prospective study. Circulation 2010;122(15):1449–55.

17. Swerdlow CD, Gunderson BD, Ousdigian KT, et al. Downloadable algorithm to reduce inappropriate shocks caused by fractures of implantable cardioverter-defibrillator leads. Circulation 2008; 118(21):2122–9.

18. Welte N, Strik M, Eschalier R, et al. Multicenter investigation of an implantable cardioverter-defibrillator algorithm to detect oversensing. Heart Rhythm 2017;14(7):1008–15.

19. Sung RK, Massie BM, Varosy PD, et al. Long-term electrical survival analysis of Riata and Riata ST silicone leads: national Veterans Affairs experience. Heart Rhythm 2012;9(12):1954–61.

20. Hauser RG, Kallinen LM, Almquist AK, et al. Early failure of a small-diameter high-voltage implantable cardioverter-defibrillator lead. Heart Rhythm 2007; 4(7):892–6.

21. Krahn AD, Champagne J, Healey JS, et al. Outcome of the Fidelis implantable cardioverter-defibrillator lead advisory: a report from the Canadian Heart Rhythm Society device advisory committee. Heart Rhythm 2008;5(5):639–42.

22. Birnie DH, Parkash R, Exner DV, et al. Clinical predictors of Fidelis lead failure: report from the Canadian Heart Rhythm Society device committee. Circulation 2012;125(10):1217–25.

23. Abdelhadi RH, Saba SF, Ellis CR, et al. Independent multicenter study of Riata and Riata ST implantable cardioverter-defibrillator leads. Heart Rhythm 2013; 10(3):361–5.

24. Swerdlow CD, Asirvatham SJ, Ellenbogen KA, et al. Troubleshooting implanted cardioverter defibrillator sensing problems I. Circ Arrhythm Electrophysiol 2014;7(6):1237–61.

25. Ellenbogen KA, Gunderson BD, Stromberg KD, et al. Performance of lead integrity alert to assist in the clinical diagnosis of implantable cardioverter defibrillator lead failures: analysis of different implantable cardioverter defibrillator leads. Circ Arrhythm Electrophysiol 2013;6(6):1169–77.

26. Hauser RG, Abdelhadi RH, McGriff DM, et al. Failure of a novel silicone-polyurethane copolymer (Optim) to prevent implantable cardioverter-defibrillator lead insulation abrasions. Europace 2013;15(2): 278–83.

27. Swerdlow CD, Kass RM, Khoynezhad A, et al. Inside-out insulation failure of a defibrillator lead with abrasion-resistant coating. Heart Rhythm 2013; 10(7):1063–6.

28. Goldstein MA, Badri M, Kocovic D, et al. Electrical failure of an ICD lead due to a presumed insulation defect only diagnosed by a maximum output shock. Pacing Clin Electrophysiol 2013;36(9):1068–71.

29. Satpathy R, Hee T, Esterbrooks D, et al. Delayed defibrillator lead perforation: an increasing phenomenon. Pacing Clin Electrophysiol 2008;31(1):10–2.

30. Laborderie J, Barandon L, Ploux S, et al. Management of subacute and delayed right ventricular perforation with a pacing or an implantable cardioverter-defibrillator lead. Am J Cardiol 2008; 102(10):1352–5.

31. Jeevanantham V, Levine E, Budzikowski AS, et al. Defibrillation coil reversal: a rare cause of abnormal noise and inappropriate shocks. Pacing Clin Electrophysiol 2008;31(3):375–7.

32. Gunderson BD, Swerdlow CD, Wilcox JM, et al. Causes of ventricular oversensing in implantable cardioverter-defibrillators: implications for diagnosis of lead fracture. Heart Rhythm 2010;7(5):626–33.

33. Verlato R, Facchin D, Catanzariti D, et al. Clinical outcomes in patients with implantable cardioverter defibrillators and Sprint Fidelis leads. Heart 2013; 99(11):799–804.

34. Steinberg C, Padfield GJ, Hahn E, et al. Lead integrity alert is useful for assessment of performance of Biotronik Linox leads. J Cardiovasc Electrophysiol 2015;26(12):1340–5.

35. Wollmann CG, Lawo T, Kuhlkamp V, et al. Implantable defibrillators with enhanced detection algorithms: detection performance and safety results from the Painfree SST study. Pacing Clin Electrophysiol 2014;37(9):1198–209.

36. Mulpuru SK, Noheria A, Cha YM, et al. Nonsustained lead noise alert associated with repeating pattern of signals on the ventricular channel: is there true concern for lead malfunction? Heart Rhythm 2014; 11(3):526–8.

37. Koneru JN, Swerdlow CD, Ploux S, et al. Mechanisms of undersensing by a noise detection

algorithm that utilizes far-field electrograms with near-field bandpass filtering. J Cardiovasc Electrophysiol 2017;28(2):224–32.

38. Chung R, Garrett PD, Wisnoskey B, et al. Clinical implications of real time implantable cardioverter-defibrillator high voltage lead short circuit detection. International Journal of Heart Rhythm 2017; 2(1):49.

39. Mizobuchi M, Enjoji Y. Successful detection of a high-energy electrical short circuit and a "rescue" shock using a novel automatic shocking-vector adjustment algorithm. HeartRhythm Case Rep 2015;1(1):27–30.

40. Ryan JD, Tempel ND, Engle DD, et al. Oversensing of transthoracic excitation stimuli in contemporary pacemakers. Pacing Clin Electrophysiol 2018; 41(3):340.

41. Nagel JH. Biopotential amplifiers. In: Bronzino JD, editor. Biomedical engineering hand book. 2nd edition. Boca Raton (FL): Springer-Verlag New York; 2000. 70.71-70.14.

42. Lakshmanadoss U, Hackett V, Deshmukh P. Externalized conductor cables in Quicksite left ventricular pacing lead and Riata right ventricular lead in a single patient: a common problem with silicone insulation. Cardiol Res 2012;3(5):230–1.

43. Mendenhall GS, Saba S. Electrical dysfunction associated with conductor externalization of a silicone left ventricular lead. Pacing Clin Electrophysiol 2015;38(3):357–61.

44. Ploux S, Varma N, Strik M, et al. Optimizing implantable cardioverter-defibrillator remote monitoring: a practical guide. JACC Clin Electrophysiol 2017; 3(4):315–28.

45. Blanck Z, Axtell K, Brodhagen K, et al. Inappropriate shocks in patients with Fidelis(R) lead fractures: impact of remote monitoring and the lead integrity algorithm. J Cardiovasc Electrophysiol 2011; 22(10):1107–14.

46. Liu J, Qin D, Rattan R, et al. Longitudinal follow-up of externalized Riata leads. Am J Cardiol 2013; 112(10):1616–8.

47. Hayes D, Freedman R, Curtis AB, et al. Prevalence of externalized conductors in Riata and Riata ST silicone leads: results from the prospective, multicenter Riata lead evaluation study. Heart Rhythm 2013;10(12):1778–82.

48. Zeitler EP, Pokorney SD, Zhou K, et al. Cable externalization and electrical failure of the Riata family of implantable cardioverter-defibrillator leads: a systematic review and meta-analysis. Heart Rhythm 2015;12(6):1233–40.

Infection Management

Daniel C. DeSimone, MD[a,b,*], Muhammad Rizwan Sohail, MD[a,b]

KEYWORDS

- Device infection • Lead extraction • Sonication • TEE • AHA guidelines

KEY POINTS

- Cardiovascular implantable electronic device (CIED) infections can be life-threatening and require complete device removal to achieve cure.
- Cultures from the device and generator pocket should be obtained in all cases of suspected infection, and the device system should undergo sonication to identify the infecting microorganism.
- Reimplantation of a new CIED should be determined in a multispecialty approach.

INTRODUCTION

Cardiovascular implantable electronic devices (CIEDs) have been available since the 1960s and have undergone significant advancement related to size, complexity, and type of generator and lead materials. Along with these manufacturing changes and improvement in implantation techniques, indications of CIED therapy for patients with heart failure and arrhythmias have continued to expand, improving quality of life and reducing mortality in device receipients.[1,2] However, the rate of CIED infection has increased along with increasing rate of CIED implantation.[1,3] Consequently, patients living with CIEDs are older with multiple comorbidities such as chronic kidney disease, diabetes mellitus, heart failure, or receiving chronic corticosteroid and oral anticoagulant therapy, putting them at higher risk of developing a CIED infection.[1,4]

EPIDEMIOLOGY

More than half a million patients undergo CIED implantation in the United States each year,[2,4] including permanent pacemakers (PPM), implantable cardioverter defibrillator (ICD), and cardiac resynchronization therapy-defibrillators (CRT-D). Rates of CIED infection vary from 0.5% to 1% for initial implantation and 1% to 5% for replacement or upgrade procedures.[1,2] CIED infection may present with infection limited to the generator pocket site, or systemic infection with lead and/or valve vegetations associated with bloodstream infection.[3]

CIED infection rates have increased out of proportion to the rate of device implantation. Device system replacement and upgrade procedures are associated with higher rates of infection compared with initial device implantation.

FINANCIAL BURDEN

According to a study by Greenspon and colleagues[4] using the Nationwide Inpatient Sample (NIS), there was an increase in cost for in-hospital charges from $75,000 in 1993 to over $146,000 by 2008. In another study using the NIS database from 2003 to 2011, an increase in hospitalization charges from $91,348 in 2003 to $173,211 in 2011 was observed.[5] In a recently published analysis of 5401 Medicare fee-for-service beneficiaries

Disclosures: Dr. M.R. Sohail reports receiving funds from TYRX Inc and Medtronic for prior research, unrelated to this article, administered according to a sponsored research agreement between Mayo Clinic and study sponsor that prospectively defined the scope of the research effort and corresponding budget; and honoraria/consulting fees from Medtronic Inc, Spectranetics, and Boston Scientific Corp. Dr D.C. DeSimone has no financial disclosure.

[a] Division of Infectious Diseases, Department of Medicine, Mayo Clinic College of Medicine and Science, 200 1st Street Southwest, Rochester, MN, USA; [b] Department of Cardiovascular Diseases, Mayo Clinic College of Medicine and Science, 200 1st Street Southwest, Rochester, MN, USA
* Corresponding author.
E-mail address: desimone.daniel@mayo.edu

cardiacEP.theclinics.com

with CIED infection in the year following implantation or upgraded CIED between 2010 and 2012, infection-related costs including extraction/replacement accounted for more than half of the expenditures for patients with surgical/hospital intervention, resulting in high health care expenditure for managing CIED infections in this population.[6] Sohail and colleagues[7] reviewed a large US payer database evaluating the costs associated with CIED infection and found a substantial increase in annual expenditures the year after implant when infection occurs.

MICROBIOLOGY

Most microorganisms (60%–80%) involved in CIED infection include staphylococcal species including *Staphylococcus aureus* and coagulase-negative staphylococci (CoNS).[3] Nonstaphylococcal causes of CIED infections include polymicrobial infections; gram-negative bacteria including *Pseudomonas aeruginosa*, *Serratia marcescens*, *Acinetobacter baumannii*, *Klebsiella pneumoniae*, and *Morganella morganii*; other gram-positive bacteria such as *Enterococcus faecalis*, *Streptococcus bovis*, *Corynebacteria* subspecies, and *Streptococcus viridans*; fungi including *Candida albicans*, *C glabrata*, *C tropicalis*, *Aspergillus* subspecies, and mycobacteria.[3,8]

Key points to know are that *S aureus* and CoNS are responsible for the majority of CIED infections, and empiric antibiotic therapy should include intravenous vancomycin to cover staphylococci.

RISK FACTORS FOR CARDIOVASCULAR IMPLANTABLE ELECTRONIC DEVICE INFECTIONS

Factors that may increase the risk of CIED infection include patient comorbidities, implanter's experience and technique, and procedural characteristics.[9] Identification of these risks factors is critical for risk stratification, modifying clinical practice, and implementing strategies such as periprocedural antimicrobial prophylaxis to reduce risk of device infection. Medical comorbidities associated with increased infection risk include diabetes mellitus, renal failure, heart failure, oral anticoagulant use, and long-term corticosteroid use.[1,9–12] Physician experience has been associated with the risk of CIED infection and mechanical complications. Physicians who implant CIEDs at low volumes compared with higher-volume implanters have higher rates of CIED infection and mechanical complications at 90 days.[13] Procedural characteristics associated with increased risk of CIED infection include fever within 24 hours

prior to implantation, use of preprocedural temporary pacing, device revision, and early repeat intervention. Administration of periprocedural antibiotic prophylaxis and implantation of a new system, compared with partial or complete system replacement, have consistently been associated with lower risk of infection.[1,14]

Key points include

- High-volume CIED implanters have lower rates of CIED infections and mechanical complications compared with lower-volume implanters.
- Renal failure, immunosuppression, and oral anticoagulant use increase risk of CIED infection.
- Use of periprocedure antibiotic prophylaxis decreases the risk of CIED infection.

PATHOGENESIS

Cardiac device generator or leads may get contaminated at the time of implantation, during manipulation of the pocket such as end-of-life battery replacement, lead revision, or if the device erodes through the skin, resulting in subsequent clinical infection. Hematogenous seeding of the CIED pocket or lead may occur because of bacteremia from a distant site of infection.[1] Interactions between the host, pathogen, and device are unique and impact bacterial adherence to the surface of the device generator and/or leads. Shape and surface properties of the device generator casing such as stainless steel or titanium, and material used for lead insulation such as polyvinyl chloride, polyethylene, polyurethane, and silicone can affect the risk of CIED infection.[1,15] Furthermore, certain bacteria, particularly staphylococci, possess adhesive surface proteins or polysaccharide capsules that coat their surface and have affinity to plastic polymers used in devices.[1]

Understanding biofilm formation and the role it plays in microbial resistance is critical in the management of CIED infection. To develop a biofilm, bacteria attach to a device and accumulate in layers forming an extracellular slime layer that firmly attaches the bacteria to each other and device. Within this matrix, the bacteria are metabolically quiescent and render themselves more resistant to antibiotics that have difficulty penetrating the biofilm and killing the metabolically inactive organisms. Moreover, bacteria are protected from host defenses within this slime layer.[1,16,17]

Key points include

- CIED pocket infections typically occur because of contamination of device during implantation or in the early postoperative period.

- CIED lead infection may occur because of extension of pocket infection or hematogenous seeding of leads from distant sources of bacteremia.
- Pocket manipulation for generator replacement or upgrades increases risk of developing a CIED infection.
- Biofilm formation on a device surface protects bacteria from antibiotic therapy and allows for persistence of bacterial infection

DIAGNOSIS AND MANAGEMENT OF CARDIOVASCULAR IMPLANTABLE ELECTRONIC DEVICE INFECTIONS

CIED infections may present with one of the following scenarios

1. Erythema at the pocket site with or without bacteremia
2. Erosion of the generator or leads through the skin
3. Bacteremia without evidence of pocket-generator site infection

CIED removal is not indicated in cases with superficial or incisional infection at the device pocket. Treatment with an oral antibiotic, with antistaphylococcal activity, for 7 to 10 days is often sufficient in these cases.[1]

In cases of established CIED generator or lead infection, complete hardware removal is mandatory to achieve cure.[1] In 1 study, early (within 3 days of presentation) extraction was shown to shorten hospital length of stay and decreased in-hospital mortality.[18] In patients in whom the device was retained (complete or partial) and placed on chronic antibiotic suppression, patients had high rates of relapse and mortality.[1,19,20]

Management of patients who present with bacteremia without evidence of pocket site infection can be challenging. In these cases, CIED may be the source of the bacteremia, or the source may be from a distant focus such as the genitourinary or respiratory tract, intra-abdominal infection, osteomyelitis, or diabetic foot ulcer. Accurately distinguishing CIED-related versus non-CIED related bacteremia can be difficult, and advanced imaging, such as PET/CT can be helpful in these complicated cases.

Fluorine 18 fluorodeoxyglucose (^{18}F-FDG) positron emission technology (PET)/computed tomography (CT) imaging has been increasingly used in the diagnosis of CIED infection. In a meta-analysis by Mahmood and colleagues,[21] the pooled sensitivity of ^{18}F-FDG PET/CT in the diagnosis of CIED infection was 83%, and pooled specificity was 89%, with higher sensitivity (96%) and specificity (97%) for diagnosing pocket infections. A major issue with ^{18}F-FDG PET/CT imaging is its high costs to perform and lack of reimbursement by insurance companies for this indication. However, unnecessary device removal is not without risk or high costs.[1,7,21] See **Fig. 1** for PET/CT imaging of a patient with a CIED infection.

A multinational survey of members from the Heart Rhythm Society, spanning 70 countries and 6 continents, suggested a wide variation in

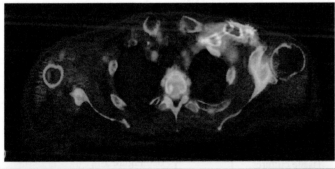
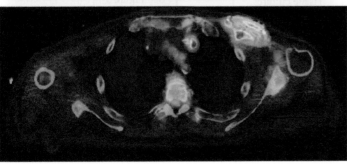

Fig. 1. PET/CT imaging in a patient with cardiovascular implantable electronic device infection. Increased FDG activity at cardiac device generator pocket site extending proximally along device leads, consistent with infection. (*Courtesy of* Mayo Foundation for Medical Education and Research, Rochester, MN; with permission. *By permission of* Mayo Foundation for Medical Education and Research. All rights reserved.)

clinical practice in managing CIED infection with significant deviations from published guidelines.[22] These data suggest that about half of the time, superficial (incisional) site infections were treated with antibiotics alone, which is consistent with the guidelines. However, two-thirds of the patients with deep pocket infections were also being managed conservatively, with antibiotics alone and without device removal, a practice known to be associated with high risk of relapse and a clear deviation from the published guidelines.[22]

The authors recommend a team-based approach with diligent discussion between specialists in infectious diseases, cardiology, electrophysiology, and cardiothoracic surgery to develop a patient-centered treatment plan in regards to timing of device removal and reimplantation.[1,2]

STEP-WISE APPROACH TO CARDIOVASCULAR IMPLANTABLE ELECTRONIC DEVICE INFECTION DIAGNOSIS AND MANAGEMENT

Obtain 2 sets of peripheral blood cultures *before* initiating empiric antibiotics for patients with systemic symptoms of infection (**Figs. 2** and **3**). For patients in whom infection is limited to the generator pocket, who have no systemic symptoms, and in whom extraction s planned in the next 24 to 48 hours, withholding antibiotics until operative pocket and device/lead cultures are obtained is preferable.

Obtain a transesophageal echocardiogram (TEE) to assess for lead and/or valve vegetation in patients with positive blood cultures. Plan complete device generator and lead removal, including abandoned leads from prior procedures. Send pocket swabs and tissue samples for Gram stain and bacterial culture and ship device generator and lead(s) in a sterile container to microbiology laboratory for sonication[23] and bacterial cultures.

Key points include

- Complete device removal is mandatory for all CIED infection.
- Sonication of the infected device generator and leads increases the chances of microorganism identification.
- Patients in whom device removal is not feasible or safe, should be managed with chronic antibiotic suppression. However, these patients have high rates of relapse.

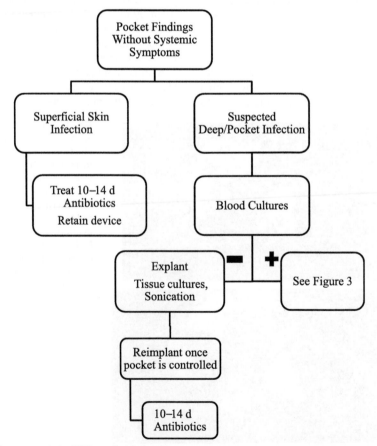

Fig. 2. Systematic approach to CIED pocket infections.

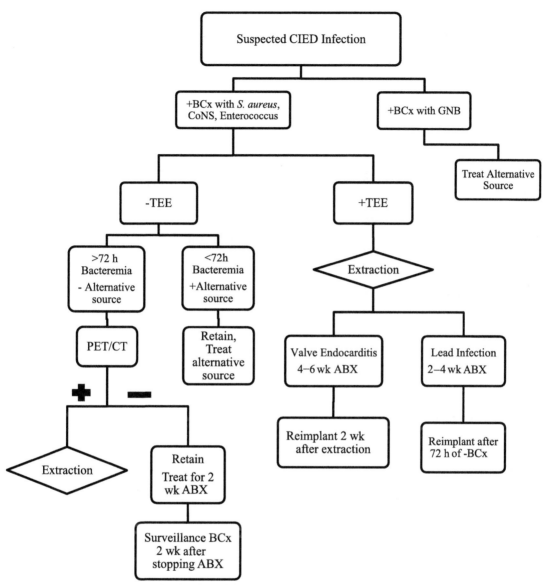

Fig. 3. Systematic approach to suspected CIED infection. BCx, blood cultures; CIED, cardiovascular implantable electronic device; CoNS, coagulase negative staphylococci; GNB, gram-negative bacteria; PET/CT, positron emission tomography/computed tomography; TEE, transesophageal echocardiogram.

TIMING OF REPEAT DEVICE IMPLANTATION

Prior to repeat device implantation, patients should be carefully assessed for the need for ongoing CIED therapy by an electrophysiologist, as up to one-third of patients no longer require a device.[1,3] In patients who present with pocket infection alone, a new device can be implanted on the contralateral side once the infected pocket has been adequately debrided. For patients who present with bloodstream infection, blood cultures should be repeated after device extraction, and a new device can be implanted if blood cultures are negative for 72 hours. Finally, for patients in whom CIED infection is complicated by infected vegetation(s) on heart valves, repeat device implantation should be delayed until after 14 days of the first negative blood culture.[1,3]

Chronic Antibiotic Suppression

There are patients with CIED infection who do not undergo complete device removal. Reasons for this may include patients who are not candidates for removal by percutaneous or surgical methods because of limited life expectancy or patient refusal for device removal.[1] These patients will often receive a 2- to 4-week course of intravenous antibiotic therapy followed by chronic antibiotic suppression. Prior published studies have shown high failure rates with this treatment approach,[24–27] which is why complete device removal is recommended for cure and lowering mortality.[3]

In a study by Tan and colleagues,[19] 660 cases of CIED infection were identified between 2005 and 2015 at the Mayo Clinic, where 48 patients were placed on chronic antibiotic suppression. Median overall survival was 1.43 years, with 18% developing relapse within 1 year. Of the patients who relapsed, approximately 33% subsequently underwent CIED extraction.[19] In a large multicenter study (MEDIC), no clinical and laboratory variables could predict successful device salvage.[28]

Key points include

- Chronic antibiotic suppression may be indicated in select patients who do not undergo complete CIED removal.
- High rates of relapse occur with chronic antibiotic suppression.

PREVENTION OF CARDIOVASCULAR IMPLANTABLE ELECTRONIC DEVICE INFECTION

Following known preventive strategies for CIED infection is crucial given the morbidity and mortality and costs associated with device infections. Several studies have examined preoperative, perioperative, and postoperative strategies to prevent CIED infection.[29] Adherence to infection control measures is critical to reduce the risk of CIED infection.[29] Preoperative strategies include nasal screening for *S aureus* and decolonization with mupirocin and chlorhexidine rinses, and a single dose of a parenteral antibiotic within 60 minutes of procedure. Intraoperative measures include skin antisepsis with chlorhexidine, pocket irrigation with normal saline, and use of an antimicrobial envelope in high-risk patients. Postoperatively, antibiotic prophylaxis should only be used if subsequent invasive manipulation of the CIED is planned. Routine use of postoperative oral antibiotic prophylaxis is unnecessary.[29]

Patients with prior history of CIED infection, device revision procedure, diabetes, and other known risk factors for CIED infection may benefit from the use of an antibiotic-impregnated envelope.[30–33] In a recent meta-analysis, use of antibiotic envelopes for CIED implantation was associated with a significantly lower rate of infection.[34]

Key points include

- Adherence to infection prevention protocols is imperative in reducing the risk of CIED infections.
- Antibiotic envelopes should be considered in patients at high risk for CIED infection.

SUMMARY

CIED infections are associated with significant morbidity and mortality for patients, and are a significant financial burden on the health care system. Early diagnosis and appropriate management with removal of infected device can be a life-saving intervention. These complicated cases are best managed with a multidisciplinary team approach. Adherence to known prevention strategies at the time of device implantation is critical.

REFERENCES

1. Baddour LM, Epstein AE, Erickson CC, et al. Update on cardiovascular implantable electronic device infections and their management: a scientific statement from the American Heart Association. Circulation 2010;121(3):458–77.
2. Lambert CT, Tarakji KG. Cardiac implantable electronic device infection. Cleve Clin J Med 2017; 84(12 Suppl 3):47–53.
3. Sohail MR, Uslan DZ, Khan AH, et al. Management and outcome of permanent pacemaker and implantable cardioverter-defibrillator infections. J Am Coll Cardiol 2007;49(18):1851–9.
4. Greenspon AJ, Patel JD, Lau E, et al. 16-year trends in the infection burden for pacemakers and implantable cardioverter-defibrillators in the United States 1993 to 2008. J Am Coll Cardiol 2011;58(10):1001–6.
5. Sridhar AR, Lavu M, Yarlagadda V, et al. Cardiac implantable electronic device-related infection and extraction trends in the U.S. Pacing Clin Electrophysiol 2017;40(3):286–93.
6. Greenspon AJ, Eby EL, Petrilla AA, et al. Treatment patterns, costs, and mortality among medicare beneficiaries with CIED infection. Pacing Clin Electrophysiol 2018. https://doi.org/10.1111/pace.13300.
7. Sohail MR, Eby EL, Ryan MP, et al. Incidence, treatment intensity, and incremental annual expenditures for patients experiencing a cardiac implantable electronic device infection: evidence from a large US payer database 1-year post implantation. Circ Arrhythm Electrophysiol 2016;9(8) [pii:e003929].
8. Viola GM, Awan LL, Ostrosky-Zeichner L, et al. Infections of cardiac implantable electronic devices: a retrospective multicenter observational study. Medicine 2012;91(3):123–30.
9. Polyzos KA, Konstantelias AA, Falagas ME. Risk factors for cardiac implantable electronic device

infection: a systematic review and meta-analysis. Europace 2015;17(5):767–77.

10. Sohail MR, Uslan DZ, Khan AH, et al. Risk factor analysis of permanent pacemaker infection. Clin Infect Dis 2007;45(2):166–73.

11. Lekkerkerker JC, van Nieuwkoop C, Trines SA, et al. Risk factors and time delay associated with cardiac device infections: Leiden device registry. Heart 2009;95(9):715–20.

12. Bloom H, Heeke B, Leon A, et al. Renal insufficiency and the risk of infection from pacemaker or defibrillator surgery. Pacing Clin Electrophysiol 2006;29(2): 142–5.

13. Al-Khatib SM, Lucas FL, Jollis JG, et al. The relation between patients' outcomes and the volume of cardioverter-defibrillator implantation procedures performed by physicians treating Medicare beneficiaries. J Am Coll Cardiol 2005;46(8):1536–40.

14. Klug D, Balde M, Pavin D, et al. Risk factors related to infections of implanted pacemakers and cardioverter-defibrillators: results of a large prospective study. Circulation 2007;116(12):1349–55.

15. Darouiche RO. Device-associated infections: a macroproblem that starts with microadherence. Clin Infect Dis 2001;33(9):1567–72.

16. Kong KF, Vuong C, Otto M. Staphylococcus quorum sensing in biofilm formation and infection. Int J Med Microbiol 2006;296(2–3):133–9.

17. Vuong C, Otto M. Staphylococcus epidermidis infections. Microbes Infect 2002;4(4):481–9.

18. Viganego F, O'Donoghue S, Eldadah Z, et al. Effect of early diagnosis and treatment with percutaneous lead extraction on survival in patients with cardiac device infections. Am J Cardiol 2012;109(10): 1466–71.

19. Tan EM, DeSimone DC, Sohail MR, et al. Outcomes in patients with cardiovascular implantable electronic device infection managed with chronic antibiotic suppression. Clin Infect Dis 2017;64(11): 1516–21.

20. Sekiguchi Y. Conservative therapy for the management of cardiac implantable electronic device infection. J Arrhythmia 2016;32(4):293–6.

21. Mahmood M, Kendi AT, Farid S, et al. Role of (18)F-FDG PET/CT in the diagnosis of cardiovascular implantable electronic device infections: a meta-analysis. J Nucl Cardiol 2017. https://doi.org/10.1007/s12350-017-1063-0.

22. DeSimone DC, Chahal AA, DeSimone CV, et al. International survey of knowledge, attitudes, and practices of cardiologists regarding prevention and management of cardiac implantable electronic device infections. Pacing Clin Electrophysiol 2017; 40(11):1260–8.

23. Nagpal A, Patel R, Greenwood-Quaintance KE, et al. Usefulness of sonication of cardiovascular implantable electronic devices to enhance microbial detection. Am J Cardiol 2015;115(7):912–7.

24. Cacoub P, Leprince P, Nataf P, et al. Pacemaker infective endocarditis. Am J Cardiol 1998;82(4): 480–4.

25. Chua JD, Wilkoff BL, Lee I, et al. Diagnosis and management of infections involving implantable electrophysiologic cardiac devices. Ann Intern Med 2000; 133(8):604–8.

26. Camus C, Leport C, Raffi F, et al. Sustained bacteremia in 26 patients with a permanent endocardial pacemaker: assessment of wire removal. Clin Infect Dis 1993;17(1):46–55.

27. del Rio A, Anguera I, Miro JM, et al. Surgical treatment of pacemaker and defibrillator lead endocarditis: the impact of electrode lead extraction on outcome. Chest 2003;124(4):1451–9.

28. Peacock JE Jr, Stafford JM, Le K, et al. Attempted salvage of infected cardiovascular implantable electronic devices: are there clinical factors that predict success? Pacing Clin Electrophysiol 2018. https://doi.org/10.1111/pace.13319.

29. Palraj BR, Farid S, Sohail MR. Strategies to prevent infections associated with cardiovascular implantable electronic devices. Expert Rev Med devices 2017;14(5):371–81.

30. Bloom HL, Constantin L, Dan D, et al. Implantation success and infection in cardiovascular implantable electronic device procedures utilizing an antibacterial envelope. Pacing Clin Electrophysiol 2011; 34(2):133–42.

31. Kolek MJ, Patel NJ, Clair WK, et al. Efficacy of a bioabsorbable antibacterial envelope to prevent cardiac implantable electronic device infections in high-risk subjects. J Cardiovasc Electrophysiol 2015;26(10):1111–6.

32. Kolek MJ, Dresen WF, Wells QS, et al. Use of an antibacterial envelope is associated with reduced cardiac implantable electronic device infections in high-risk patients. Pacing Clin Electrophysiol 2013; 36(3):354–61.

33. Henrikson CA, Sohail MR, Acosta H, et al. Antibacterial envelope is associated with low infection rates after implantable cardioverter-defibrillator and cardiac resynchronization therapy device replacement: results of the citadel and centurion studies. JACC Clin Electrophysiol 2017;3(10):1158–67.

34. Koerber SM, Turagam MK, Winterfield J, et al. Use of antibiotic envelopes to prevent cardiac implantable electronic device infections: a meta-analysis. J Cardiovasc Electrophysiol 2018. https://doi.org/10.1111/jce.13436.

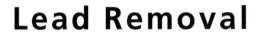

Lead Removal

Nomenclature, Definitions, and Metrics of Cardiovascular Implantable Electronic Device Lead Management

Bruce L. Wilkoff, MD, FHRS, CCDS

KEYWORDS

- Transvenous lead extraction • Outcomes • Complications • Definitions • Pacemaker
- Implantable defibrillator

KEY POINTS

- Quality and quality improvement are dependent on specific definitions and accurate calculation of metrics of success, failure, and complications.
- Transparency of volume and outcomes on a center- and operator-specific basis is required and provides the foundation for communication in the literature and to patients.
- Extraction programs and operator-specific information on volume, clinical success rates, and complication rates for lead removal and extraction should be available and discussed with the patient before any lead removal procedure.
- Participation in a registry, either center specific or as part of a multicenter effort, provides for benchmarks of quality and is the cornerstone of a quality lead management program.

INTRODUCTION

The most effective tool in advancing quality patient care is consistent nomenclature and measurement of outcomes, success and failure, and complications. Transparency is challenging to the individual physician and also to the institutions within which physicians labor. In the early days of transvenous lead extraction there were few tools, poorly defined techniques, and few practitioners. However, there was a strong commitment to solving a clinical problem and continuous quality improvement. There was a collaborative and voluntary registry, the Cook Extraction Registry, dominated by a handful of brave extractors who labored to define the tools, techniques, success, and failures.[1,2] This article describes the current definitions, metrics of outcomes, and standards for care worldwide that have evolved from this initial effort.

DEFINITIONS AND METRICS

There are three distinct aspects to every task: (1) goal or indication, (2) process or technique, and (3) evaluation or measures of achieving the goal thus resolving the indicated condition. This third aspect of procedural definition and the derived metrics determine the success, failure, and quality of the process. This is highly dependent on the specificity of the nomenclature and definitions, and measurable and quantifiable outcomes. Interpretation of the literature, its application to hospital- or physician-specific outcomes, and simple

Disclosure Statement: Consultant: Medtronic, Abbott, Spectranetics.
Robert and Suzanne Tomsich Department of Cardiovascular Medicine, Cardiac Pacing and Tachyarrhythmia Devices, Sydell and Arnold Miller Family Heart and Vascular Institute, Cleveland Clinic, 9500 Euclid Avenue, Desk J2-2, Cleveland, OH 44022, USA
E-mail address: wilkofb@ccf.org

Card Electrophysiol Clin 10 (2018) 609–613
https://doi.org/10.1016/j.ccep.2018.08.001

assessment and communication of risk and benefit to the patient depends on the words and definitions, consistently applied. The definitions and metrics described in this article are derived from the three North American Society for Pacing and Electrophysiology Heart Rhythm Society consensus documents from 2000, 2009, and 2017.[3–5] Unfortunately not all of the literature has used these descriptors and extreme care must be taken when interpreting reported results. These definitions have also been used by the European Heart Rhythm Society in their publications with some modifications in the training requirements.[6,7] The most recent consensus statement represented all four continental heart rhythm societies (Heart Rhythm Society, European Heart Rhythm Association, Asian Pacific Heart Rhythm Society Latin American Heart Rhythm Society) and the North American societies representing cardiology, cardiothoracic surgery, anesthesiology, and infectious disease. Up until the publication of this most recent international consensus document, it was encouraged but optional to keep track of volume, outcomes, and quality. The ability to have shared decision making based on accurate knowledge of measured outcomes now requires use of this 2017 class I recommendation.

Class I Recommendation

Extraction programs and operator-specific information on volume, clinical success rates, and complication rates for lead removal and extraction should be available and discussed with the patient prior to any lead removal procedure.[5]

Although the data collection method is not prescribed, with this mandate, all lead extraction programs must collect and provide complete data transparency when communicating with patients and all other stakeholders. Shared decision making is also specifically prescribed for several conditions in the consensus statement, making use of the definitions and these metrics mandatory.

Class IIb Recommendation

Lead removal may be considered in the setting of normally functioning nonrecalled pacing or defibrillation leads for selected patients after a shared decision-making process.[5]

It is worth quoting precisely the language of the consensus document to give the sense and strength of this recommendation from this worldwide and multidisciplinary consensus statement. Throughout the document, the risk, success, safety, and the decisions made to extract or the choice of alternative techniques are dependent on these metrics and definitions.

Lead extraction program-specific success and failure metrics should be prospectively collected and communicated to patients during the decision and consent process prior to each potential lead extraction procedure. Information discussed with patients during the shared decision-making process should at least include (1) the annual lead extraction volume at that center, (2) the lead extraction clinical success rate, and (3) major procedure-related complication/death rates during hospitalization. Writing committee members firmly believe this information should be made publicly available and should be communicated to patients during the shared decision-making and informed consent process to ensure complete transparency. Additional information is likely to be valuable to the patient, including (1) personal lead extraction volume and personal number of leads removed during lead extraction procedures (yearly and lifetime), clinical success rate, and complication rate; (2) volume broken down between ICD and pacing leads; and (3) extraction indications (eg, infection, lead malfunction, and superfluous leads). More complete data collection is desirable and useful to promote quality outcomes and identify opportunities for process improvement but is not required.[5]

Definitions of Lead Status

There is no formal definition of an active lead or functional lead except through inference. Therefore, an active lead is a lead that is connected to a Cardiovascular Implantable Electronic Device (CIED). A functional lead is a lead that is usable, whether abandoned or connected to a CIED.

Abandoned lead
A functional or nonfunctional lead that is left in place and is not connected to the CIED.

Nonfunctional lead
A lead that is not usable because of electrical dysfunction, regardless of whether or not it is connected to the CIED.

Definitions of Lead Removal or Extraction

The associated risk, ease or difficulty of lead removal, or descriptions of experience are highly dependent on these definitions. When very young leads are included in the denominator then the experience tends to be overstated and the outcomes not reflective of the skill, safety, or outcomes or reflect the tools required. Even when these definitions are applied, many lead extractions reflect a relative lack of intravascular fibrosis and can give a false sense of how significant this procedure can become. One can also define an equation that can help in discussions of extraction experiences:

Lead removal procedures = Lead explant procedures + Lead extraction procedures.

Lead removal procedure
A procedure involving the removal of a pacing or defibrillator lead using any technique, regardless of time since implantation.

Lead explant procedure
Lead removal procedure where all leads were removed without tools or with implantation stylets and all removed leads were implanted for less than 1 year.

Lead extraction
Lead removal procedure where at least one lead removal required the assistance of equipment not typically used during lead implantation or at least one lead was implanted for greater than 1 year.

Definitions of Success and Failure

Success and failure are determined clinically and radiographically and is expressed either as a rate with the denominator of either the number of patient procedures or leads attempted for removal during a procedure.

Complete procedural success
Lead extraction procedure with removal of all targeted leads and all lead material from the vascular space, with the absence of any permanently disabling complication or procedure-related death.

Complete procedural success rate
Extraction procedures where there is complete procedural success/total number of extraction procedures.

Clinical success
Lead extraction procedures with removal of all targeted leads and lead material from the vascular space or retention of a small portion of the lead (<4 cm) that does not negatively impact the outcome goals of the procedure.

Clinical success rate
Extraction procedures where there is clinical success/total number of extraction procedures.

Failure lead extraction
Procedures in which complete procedural or clinical success cannot be achieved, or the development of any permanently disabling complication, or procedure-related death.

Failure rate
Failed extraction procedures/total number of extraction procedures. Lead removal with clinical success. Leads with attempted removal where the entire lead is taken out of the body or with retention of a small portion of the lead material (<4 cm) that does not negatively impact the outcome goals of the procedure.

Lead removal with clinical success rate
Number of leads removed with clinical success during a lead extraction/total number of leads with attempted removal.

Definitions of Infection

Isolated generator pocket infection
Localized erythema, swelling, pain, tenderness, warmth, or drainage with negative blood cultures.

Isolated pocket erosion
Device and/or leads are through the skin, with exposure of the generator or leads, with or without local signs of infection.

Bacteremia
Positive blood cultures with or without systemic infection symptoms and signs.

Pocket site infection with bacteremia
Local infection signs and positive blood cultures.

Lead infection
Lead vegetation and positive blood cultures.

Pocket site infection with lead/valvular endocarditis
Local signs and positive blood cultures and lead or valvular vegetation

CIED endocarditis without pocket infection
Positive blood cultures and lead or valvular vegetation

Occult bacteremia with probable CIED infection
Absence of alternative source, resolves after CIED extraction.

Situations in which CIED infection is not certain
Impending exteriorization, isolated left heart valvular endocarditis in a patient with a CIED.

Table 1 Complications	
Major	0.19%–1.80%
Death	0.19%–1.20%
Cardiac avulsion	0.19%–0.96%
Vascular laceration	0.16%–0.41%
Respiratory arrest	0.20%
Cerebrovascular accident	0.07%–0.08%
Pericardial effusion requiring intervention	0.23%–0.59%
Hemothorax requiring intervention	0.07%–0.20%
Cardiac arrest	0.07%
Thromboembolism requiring intervention	0.07%
Flail tricuspid valve leaflet requiring intervention	0.03%
Massive pulmonary embolism	0.08%
Minor	0.60%–6.20%
Pericardial effusion without intervention	0.07%–0.16%
Hematoma requiring evacuation	0.90%–1.60%
Venous thrombosis requiring medical intervention	0.10%–0.21%
Vascular repair at venous entry site	0.07%–0.13%
Migrated lead fragment without sequelae	0.20%
Bleeding requiring blood transfusion	0.08%–1.00%
Arteriovenous fistula requiring intervention	0.16%
Coronary sinus dissection	0.13%
Pneumothorax requiring chest tube	1.10%
Worsening tricuspid valve function	0.32%–0.59%
Pulmonary embolism	0.24%–0.59%

Data from Refs.[9–15]

Superficial incisional infection

Involves only skin and subcutaneous tissue of the incision, not the deep soft tissues (eg, fascia and/or muscle) of the incision.

BENCHMARKS

The second component of risk assessment includes an understanding of acceptable standards for quality. The success, failure, and complication rates need to be placed into context (**Table 1**). The ranges of the benchmarks and the quality of the benchmarks will improve as public reporting of individual and center data is more common.[8] The clinical success rates should exceed 95% and are often greater than 98%.

DATA MANAGEMENT

The cornerstone of quality is consistent tracking of outcomes. This is completely dependent on carefully applied nomenclature and metrics. Even though the method of obtaining or validating the statistics was not prescribed, it was the strong opinion of the lead management document writers that all centers performing lead extraction procedures maintain or participate in a multicenter data capture system. They go on to say that the ability to calculate site-specific metrics for procedural success, procedural failure, and complications for all lead removal procedures was crucial. They endorsed the previously described definitions to provide standardization of the data.

Capture of these statistics provides the most important opportunity for outcome of process improvement based on periodic review of complications. This mechanism provides continuous commitment to quality improvement. Data to be included in these data repositories include:

1. Patient demographic information
2. Operator information
3. Indications for extraction (eg, infection, lead malfunction, and superfluous leads)
4. Type of lead removed (implantable cardioverter-defibrillator vs pacing)
5. Lead extraction clinical success rates
6. Procedure success rates (complete and clinical)
7. Major and minor complications
8. Deaths that occur during the procedure or within the early or late post-procedure phases

There are two current multicenter registries. These provide some opportunity for benchmarks and ongoing center specific data collection. However, the responsibility comes down to the individual extraction program and transvenous lead extraction operator.

1. The European Society of Cardiology–sponsored European Lead Extraction ConTRolled Registry has yielded important results that can serve as benchmarks for clinical success rates, complication rates, and mortality using the definitions from the 2009 Heart Rhythm Society Extraction document: www.escardio.org/Subspecialtycommunities/European-Heart-Rhythm-Association-(EHRA)/partner-organisationsnetworks/ELECTRa-Registry.[7]

2. The Extract Registry and Study Group currently has six centers in the United States and one in Australia and is actively recruiting additional centers: http://www.extractstudygroup.org

SUMMARY

Transvenous lead extraction has matured significantly as a discipline since the late 1980s. Most of this development is attributable to the commitment to quality anchored by accurately defining and consistent reporting of outcomes. It is only by consistent use of these definitions; calculation of the success, failure, and complication rates; and the willingness to be transparent about these results that physicians can continue to improve this important part of patient care.

REFERENCES

1. Fearnot NE, Smith HJ, Goode LB, et al. Intravascular lead extraction using locking stylets, sheaths, and other techniques. Pacing Clin Electrophysiol 1990; 13(12 Pt 2):1864–70.
2. Smith HJ, Fearnot NE, Byrd CL, et al. Five-years experience with intravascular lead extraction. U.S. lead extraction database. Pacing Clin Electrophysiol 1994;17(11 Part II):2016–20.
3. Love CJ, Wilkoff BL, Byrd CL, et al. Recommendations for extraction of chronically implanted transvenous pacing and defibrillator leads: indications, facilities, training. Pacing Clin Electrophysiol 2000; 23:544–51.
4. Wilkoff BL, Love CJ, Byrd CL, et al. Transvenous lead extraction: heart rhythm society expert consensus on facilities, training, indications, and patient management: this document was endorsed by the American Heart Association (AHA). Heart Rhythm 2009;6:1085–104.
5. Kusumoto FM, Schoenfeld MH, Wilkoff BL, et al. HRS expert consensus statement on cardiovascular implantable electronic device lead management and extraction. Heart Rhythm 2017;14(12):e503–51.
6. Deharo JC, Bongiorni MG, Rozkovec A, et al. Pathways for training and accreditation for transvenous lead extraction: a European Heart Rhythm Association position paper. Europace 2012;14(1):124–34.
7. Bongiorni MG, Kennergren C, Butter C, et al, ELECTRa Investigators. The European Lead Extraction ConTRolled (ELECTRa) study: a European Heart Rhythm Association (EHRA) registry of transvenous lead extraction outcomes. Eur Heart J 2017;38(40): 2995–3005.
8. Wazni O, Epstein LM, Carrillo RG, et al. Lead extraction in the contemporary setting: the lexicon study: an observational retrospective study of consecutive laser lead extractions. J Am Coll Cardiol 2010;55: 579–86.
9. Brunner MP, Cronin EM, Jacob J, et al. Transvenous extraction of implantable cardioverter-defibrillator leads under advisory: a comparison of Riata, Sprint Fidelis, and non-recalled implantable cardioverter-defibrillator leads. Heart Rhythm 2013;10:1444–50.
10. Ji SY, Gundewar S, Palma EC. Subclavian venoplasty may reduce implant times and implant failures in the era of increasing device upgrades. Pacing Clin Electrophysiol 2012;35:444–8.
11. Pokorney SD, Zhou K, Matchar DB, et al. Optimal management of Riata leads with no known electrical abnormalities or externalization: a decision analysis. J Cardiovasc Electrophysiol 2015;26:184–91.
12. Priori SG, Auricchio A, Nisam S, et al. To replace or not to replace: a systematic approach to respond to device advisories. J Cardiovasc Electrophysiol 2009;20:164–70.
13. Hamid S, Arujuna A, Khan S, et al. Extraction of chronic pacemaker and defibrillator leads from the coronary sinus: laser infrequently used but required. Europace 2009;11:213–5.
14. Shepherd E, Stuart G, Martin R, et al. Extraction of SelectSecure leads compared to conventional pacing leads in patients with congenital heart disease and congenital atrioventricular block. Heart Rhythm 2015;12:1227–32.
15. Sridhar AR, Lavu M, Yarlagadda V, et al. Cardiac implantable electronic device-related infection and extraction trends in the U.S. Pacing Clin Electrophysiol 2017;40:286–93.

Anesthesia Considerations for Lead Extraction

Matthew Fischer, MD[a], Reed Harvey, MD[a], Noel G. Boyle, MD, PhD[b], Jonathan K. Ho, MD[a],*

KEYWORDS

- Anesthesiology • Lead extraction • Laser lead extraction • Perioperative management

KEY POINTS

- Anesthesiologists possess both an intimate knowledge of the operative environment and an expertise in perioperative management of high-risk patients and procedures. The anesthesia team should be engaged in perioperative planning and development of institutional practices for lead extraction.
- Preoperative preparation involves assessment of patient risk, selection of operative venue, and coordination of resources to support the procedure.
- Intraoperative anesthetic management may vary, but typically includes general anesthesia with an endotracheal tube, invasive arterial pressure monitoring, adequate volume access for resuscitation, echocardiographic monitoring, preparation for blood transfusion, and initiation of cardiopulmonary bypass.
- The postoperative management is determined largely by preexisting patient factors as well as the occurrence of significant intraoperative complications.

After the decision to proceed with lead extraction is made, the anesthesiologist becomes an integral part of the perioperative team and plays a pivotal role in caring for these patients. Anesthetic management of lead extractions focuses on maintaining patient comfort, providing optimal operating conditions, and ensuring patient safety. Safety and risk reduction is of particular importance in lead extraction cases because of the severity of potential complications, which may require emergent surgical intervention. Ensuring patient safety requires a thorough preoperative evaluation and risk assessment, development of a comprehensive intraoperative plan to account for infrequent but life-threatening complications, and coordination of appropriate postoperative care. The operative team can include cardiologists/ cardiac electrophysiologists, cardiac surgeons, anesthesiologists, perfusionists, nurses from multiple care areas, radiation technologists, and industry representatives. With such a large team, effective communication is essential in all phases of care because each team member plays a critical role in a successful and safe extraction procedure.

PREOPERATIVE CONSIDERATIONS AND PLANNING

As the implant rate of cardiovascular implantable electronic devices (CIED) continues to grow, so too does the rate of CIED-related complications and the need for lead removal or extraction.[1–3]As defined by both the 2009 and 2017 Heart Rhythm Society's expert consensus statements, lead

---

Disclosure Statement: None.

[a] Department of Anesthesiology and Perioperative Medicine, UCLA Health System, David Geffen School of Medicine at UCLA, Ronald Reagan UCLA Medical Center, 757 Westwood Plaza, Suite 3325, Los Angeles, CA 90095, USA; [b] Department of Medicine, UCLA Health System, David Geffen School of Medicine at UCLA, 100 UCLA Medical Plaza, Suite 660, Los Angeles, CA 90095-1679, USA

* Corresponding author.

E-mail address: jkho@mednet.ucla.edu

Card Electrophysiol Clin 10 (2018) 615–624

https://doi.org/10.1016/j.ccep.2018.04.003

extraction refers to the removal of a lead that has been implanted for more than 1 year, or a lead regardless of age that requires the assistance of specialized equipment for removal, and/or a lead from a route other than via the implant vein.[4,5] This specialized equipment refers to a wide range of devices including traction devices, such as locking stylets, mechanical cutting sheaths, laser sheaths, and electrosurgical sheaths. Although complication and mortality rates of lead extraction continue to decline with increasing operator experience and technological advances in extraction equipment, the procedure nonetheless carries significant risk to the patient. A large, multicenter observational study of pacemaker and implantable cardioverter-defibrillator (ICD) lead extraction procedures found a major complication rate of only 1.4% and mortality of 0.3%[3]; however, these rates can be much higher in some patient populations, such as those with device-related infections.[6] Cumulative mortality rates following lead extraction can range from 2.1% to 3.3% at 30 days and 8.4% to 10% at 1 year.[5] **Table 1** contains a near comprehensive list of major and minor complications associated with lead extraction procedures, as compiled by the Heart Rhythm Society. A coordinated and multidisciplinary approach involving a trained and experienced extraction team is of paramount importance in ensuring successful outcomes, minimizing complications, and responding to potentially catastrophic emergencies. The preoperative role of the anesthesiologist begins with a thorough review of the patient's history with a specific focus on the following:

- Indications for and date of device implantation
- Indications for device explantation
- Type of device (pacemaker vs defibrillator)
- Number, age, and location of leads
- Review of recent device interrogation with focus on device settings, pacemaker dependence, and history of treated malignant arrhythmias
- Review of preoperative imaging focused on identification of high-risk characteristics, such as extravascular location of leads, cardiac perforation, degree of vascular fibrosis or calcification, presence of pleural or pericardial effusions, and vascular stenosis or abnormalities
- Review of preoperative echocardiography with specific focus on ventricular function, presence of intracardiac shunts, location and course of intracardiac leads, presence of lead- or valve-associated vegetations or thrombi, and tricuspid valve regurgitation/stenosis

Table 1
Major and minor complications of lead extraction

Complications	Incidence
Major	**0.19%–1.80%**
Death	0.19%–1.20%
Cardiac avulsion	0.19%–0.96%
Vascular laceration	0.16%–0.41%
Respiratory arrest	0.20%
Cerebrovascular accident	0.07%–0.08%
Pericardial effusion requiring intervention	0.23%–0.59%
Hemothorax requiring intervention	0.07%–0.20%
Cardiac arrest	0.07%
Thromboembolism requiring intervention	0.07%
Flail tricuspid valve leaflet requiring intervention	0.03%
Massive pulmonary embolism	0.08%
Minor	**0.60%–6.20%**
Pericardial effusion without intervention	0.07%–0.16%
Hematoma requiring evacuation	0.90%–1.60%
Venous thrombosis requiring medical intervention	0.10%–0.21%
Vascular repair at venous entry site	0.07%–0.13%
Migrated lead fragment without sequelae	0.20%
Bleeding requiring blood transfusion	0.08%–1.00%
Arteriovenous fistula requiring intervention	0.16%
Coronary sinus dissection	0.13%
Pneumothorax requiring chest tube	1.10%
Worsening tricuspid valve function	0.32%–0.59%
Pulmonary embolism	0.24%–0.59%

Adapted from Kusumoto FM, Schoenfeld MH, Wilkoff BL, et al. 2017 HRS expert consensus statement on cardiovascular implantable electronic device lead management and extraction. Heart Rhythm 2017;14(12):e504–51; with permission.

- Review of cardiovascular comorbid conditions and prior cardiac surgical procedures
- Review of perioperative management of anticoagulants
- Review of a complete set of recent laboratory measurements including complete blood

count, comprehensive metabolic panel, complete coagulation panel, and blood cultures (if CIED infection is suspected or confirmed)

Although extensive planning and coordination with the patient, cardiac surgeon, and cardiac electrophysiologist has typically already taken place by the time an anesthesiologist is involved in the case, it is nonetheless critical for the anesthesiologist to review the entire patient history in creating an optimal anesthetic plan. In some low-risk cases of lead removal (eg, removal of leads less than 1 year old), monitored anesthesia care and sedation may be appropriate. In all cases of lead extraction (leads >1 year old or potential need for use of specialized equipment), general endotracheal anesthesia is indicated. General anesthesia increases the safety of the procedure

by ensuring a motionless patient with optimal surgical conditions for the operator, by allowing continuous transesophageal echocardiographic (TEE) monitoring, and by facilitating the fastest possible conversion to emergent sternotomy in the case of catastrophic vascular or cardiac injury.

Preoperative identification of risk factors that make procedural complications more likely may influence the anesthesiologist's planned vascular access, use of invasive monitors, and need for inotropic infusions. A review of high-risk characteristics associated with procedure-related complications and mortality can be found in **Table 2**. Although the risk factors for mortality in patients undergoing lead extraction are known, there are no widely adopted and validated clinical decision-making tools for predicting complications and mortality. Of particular importance to

---

Table 2
Factors associated with extraction procedure complications and longer-term mortality

Factor	Associated Risk
Age	1.05-fold ↑mortality
Female sex	4.5-fold ↑ risk of major complications
Low body mass index (<25 kg/m²)	1.8-fold ↑ risk of 30-d mortality ↑ number of procedure-related complications
History of cerebrovascular accident	2-fold ↑ risk of major complications
Severe LV dysfunction	2-fold ↑ risk of major complications
Advanced HF	1.3-to 8.5-fold ↑ risk of 30-d mortality 3-fold ↑ 1-y mortality
Renal dysfunction	ESRD: 4.8-fold ↑ risk of 30-d mortality Cr ≥2.0: ↑in-hospital mortality and 2-fold ↑ risk of 1-y mortality
Diabetes mellitus	↑ in-hospital mortality 1.71-fold ↑ mortality
Platelet count	Low platelet count: 1.7-fold ↑ risk of major complications
Coagulopathy	Elevated INR: 2.7-fold ↑ risk of major complications and 1.3-fold ↑ risk of 30-d mortality Anticoagulant use: 1.8-fold ↑ 1-y mortality
Anemia	3.3-fold ↑ risk of 30-d mortality
Number of leads extracted	3.5-fold ↑ risk of any complication 1.6-fold ↑ risk of any complication
Presence of dual-coil ICD	2.7-fold ↑ risk of 30-d mortality
Extraction for infection	2.7-to 30-fold ↑ risk of 30-d mortality 5-to 9.7-fold↑ 1-y mortality CRP >72 mg/L associated with ↑30-d mortality 3.52-fold ↑ mortality
Operator experience	2.6-fold ↑ number of procedure-related complications
Prior open heart surgery	↓ risk of major complications

Abbreviations: Cr, creatinine; CRP, C-reactive protein; ESRD, end-stage renal disease; HF, heart failure; INR, international normalized ratio; LV, left ventricle.

Adapted from Kusumoto FM, Schoenfeld MH, Wilkoff BL, et al. 2017 HRS expert consensus statement on cardiovascular implantable electronic device lead management and extraction. Heart Rhythm 2017;14(12):e504–51; with permission.

the anesthesiologist, predictors of complications during lead extraction are different from predictors of 30-day all-cause mortality, the latter being more significantly influenced by factors associated with advanced patient morbidity.[7] This difference is highlighted in patients with device-related infections. In these patients, lead explant may be less technically challenging and have a lower rate of complications due to the infection-related debridement of scar tissue surrounding the lead[8]; however, these patients are often more debilitated and have higher 30-day mortality rates.[7] A retrospective review of more than 5000 lead extractions was performed at a single center where multivariate predictors of all-cause 30-day mortality included body mass index (BMI) <25 kg/m^2, end-stage renal disease, higher NYHA functional class, lower hemoglobin, higher international normalized ratio (INR), lead extraction for infection, and extraction of a dual-coil ICD lead.[9] Although identifying sicker patients with an increased risk of poor outcomes is important, identification of characteristics associated with procedural complications and an increased need for emergency surgical intervention is more critical to the anesthesiologist. This information can assist in guiding intraoperative management, in selecting an appropriate intraoperative setting (electrophysiology laboratory vs operating room), and in determining the level of cardiac surgical involvement (scrubbed into case vs immediately available on site). In a review of patients requiring emergent surgical intervention during lead extraction, the investigators found that longer lead implant duration, the use of powered sheaths, and use of the femoral approach for extraction (likely a surrogate for a technically difficult procedure) were significantly associated with catastrophic procedural complications.[10] Prior studies have also associated a BMI less than 25 kg/m^2,[3] female sex,[11] an increased number of explanted leads,[8] and explant of dual-coil ICD leads[12,13] with procedural complications.

The presence of a preoperative prediction algorithm or score would be potentially beneficial to the anesthesiologist in creating a heightened awareness and preparedness for potential catastrophic intraoperative complications. Although a widely used and validated score for prediction of adverse procedural events does not currently exist, Bontempi and colleagues[14,15] did create and validate the lead extraction difficulty (LED) score. The LED score was calculated as follows: number of leads to be extracted + lead age (years from implant) + 1 if dual-coil/−1 if confirmed vegetation on the lead. An LED score greater than 10 was used to identify cases with long fluoroscopic time (>31.2 minutes) as a surrogate for a technically challenging procedure. Although no conclusions could be drawn between the LED score and procedural complications, the anesthesiologist's understanding and identification of factors that contribute to technical challenges can help increase preparedness and may potentially mitigate some risk.

In addition to a review of the patient's history, it is essential for the anesthesiologist to speak directly with the cardiac electrophysiologist and cardiac surgeon before the procedure to further enumerate and anticipate patient-specific concerns and to review together the procedural plan. Patients with a prior sternotomy merit special consideration in planning for safe transition to cardiopulmonary bypass in emergent situations.

Beyond anticipating and preparing for major procedural complications, the anesthesiologist must consider many other facets of the patient's history for optimal preoperative planning. Patients with decompensated heart failure, severely impaired ventricular function, or severe valvular abnormalities may require the intraoperative administration of inotropic medications for maintenance of hemodynamic stability. The anesthesiologist must be prepared for this eventuality and ensure the immediate availability of inotropes and appropriate vascular access for their administration.

As CIED infection is the leading indication for device explant, many patients may present with bacteremia and sepsis. The anesthesiologist should be aware of any positive blood cultures, current antibiotics, and any recent consultation of infectious disease specialists. It is important to discuss the perioperative timing of intravenous antibiotics with the surgical team, because their administration before device explant may influence bacterial culture results. In patients with infection, the timing and necessity of device reimplantation should be discussed with the cardiology team preoperatively.

In pacemaker-dependent patients, a plan for temporary pacing needs to be formulated in conjunction with the cardiac electrophysiologist before starting the procedure. In most cases at the authors' institution, the cardiologist uses a transvenous lead inserted via the right internal jugular vein, fixed in the basal right ventricular (RV) septum (away from the leads to be extracted), and connected to an externalized pacemaker generator.[16] This may be left in place until reimplantation can be undertaken and allows the patient to be mobile and monitored outside of an intensive care unit (ICU) setting. Patients with a history of malignant arrhythmias who require explant of an ICD will need continuous postoperative electrocardiographic (ECG) monitoring until the ICD can be safely reimplanted. Although responsibility for the long-term postoperative care of the patient will ultimately fall to the patient's primary team, this planning should nonetheless be discussed before definitive device explant.

In addition, preoperative review of the most recent echocardiographic images can assist in procedural planning and intraoperative management. Identification of large (>2.5 cm) lead- or valve-associated vegetations or thrombi should be discussed with the multidisciplinary team and may necessitate a staged approach for device explant or a device explant combined with an open cardiac surgical procedure (**Fig. 1**). In the case of large vegetations, Patel and colleagues[17] reported the safe and effective use of AngioVac for debulking before definitive device explant. The presence of severe tricuspid regurgitation (TR), especially with associated annular dilation, should be discussed preoperatively with the cardiac surgeon. Nazmul and colleagues[18] reported no improvement in the severity of symptomatic TR after percutaneous RV lead extraction (**Fig. 2**). These patients may benefit from an open lead extraction with concomitant tricuspid valve annuloplasty. An ECG may also identify the presence of intracardiac shunts (patent foramen ovale, atrial septal defect, ventricular septal defect) that increase the risk of paradoxical embolism of lead-associated vegetations/thrombi during extraction. Identification of these shunts merits discussion with the entire care team, because the patient may benefit from a percutaneously deployed occluder device before lead extraction (**Fig. 3**).

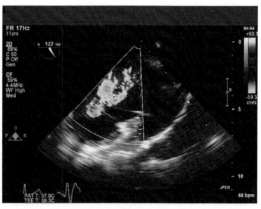

Fig. 2. Severe tricuspid regurgitation in the setting of lead-associated vegetation.

Many patients undergoing CIED extraction will be receiving therapeutic oral anticoagulation or dual antiplatelet therapy at the time of the procedure. Life-threatening hemorrhagic events are a realistic complication of device explantation. As stated previously, an elevated INR at the time of lead extraction was found to be an independent predictor of 30-day mortality.[9] The anesthesiologist should review any anticoagulant medications the patient may have been receiving preoperatively, including last date taken and associated laboratory coagulation abnormalities, and ensure that an appropriate patient-specific risk benefit discussion regarding the perioperative cessation of anticoagulants has occurred.

Intraoperative prompt recognition and management of life-threatening complications during lead extraction procedures depends primarily on

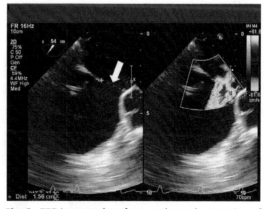

Fig. 3. TEE image taken from a planned extraction of a dual chamber device with RV lead-associated vegetations. The case was postponed because of identification of a previously undiagnosed 1.5 cm secundum ASD (*white arrow*). The patient underwent percutaneous device closure of ASD on a later date before successful lead extraction. ASD, atrial septal defect.

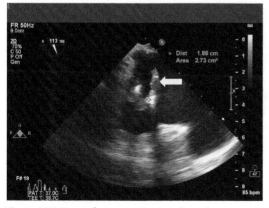

Fig. 1. TEE image from a patient undergoing percutaneous lead extraction demonstrating a 1.86 cm, mobile lead-associated vegetation (*white arrow*).

thorough, collaborative preoperative planning. The close coordination and communication between electrophysiologists, cardiac surgeons, anesthesiologists, perfusionists, and nurses, often far in advance of the planned procedure, is of the utmost importance in the execution of a safe and successful lead extraction.

INTRAOPERATIVE MANAGEMENT

After careful preoperative review of the patient's medical history, the perioperative plan is executed on the day of the procedure. In the preoperative area, the anesthesiologist performs a history and physical examination and reviews the patient's NPO status, allergies, laboratories, and availability of blood products. Specific considerations include the patient's last dose of anticoagulants, platelet count, and INR. If the lead extraction is to be performed because of an infectious process, the patient should be reassessed for signs of sepsis on the day of the procedure. In addition, the

pacemaker or ICD should be interrogated if no interrogation has been performed recently. The anesthesiologist should review whether the device is functioning properly and if the patient is pacemaker dependent.[19] ICD devices will also need to have their tachyarrhythmia therapies programmed off before the procedure. This is typically performed in the operating room after external defibrillation patches have been applied.

The anesthetic management of patients undergoing lead extraction is tailored to each patient and his/her specific risk profile. Although many lead explants are safely performed in electrophysiology laboratories, high-risk lead extractions should be performed in a hybrid operating room or interventional suite capable of facilitating a cardiopulmonary bypass machine and cardiac surgery.[19–21] An overview of the intraoperative workflow for patients undergoing laser lead extraction can be seen in **Fig. 4**.[20] Important surgical concerns for performing lead extractions in interventional suites include limitations in

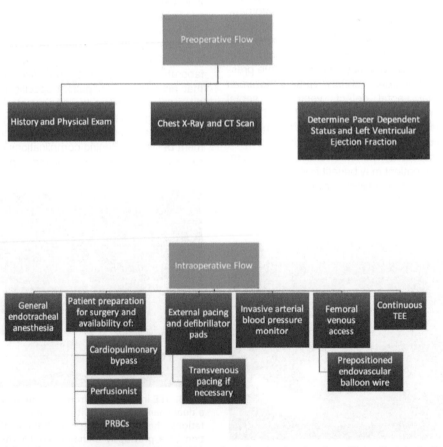

Fig. 4. Workflow for perioperative care of patients undergoing lead extraction. (*From* Fermin L, Gebhard R, Azarrafiy R, et al. Pearls of wisdom for high-risk laser lead extractions: a focused review. AnesthAnalg 2017;10:1–7; with permission.)

manipulating bed position, working around a C-arm, and possible sterility concerns. As soon as the patient is moved to the operating room or procedure table, standard ASA monitors are applied to the patient. A radial arterial line can be placed before or after induction of general anesthesia depending on whether it is needed for hemodynamic management during induction of anesthesia. Invasive hemodynamic monitoring is necessary to quickly identify acute hemodynamic decompensation as well as to guide resuscitation.[19–21] **Fig. 5** shows an example of rapid hemodynamic decompensation due to a large right atrial laceration that was quickly identified with continuous invasive blood pressure measurement.

Some lead explants may be performed under monitored anesthesia care (MAC) in suitable patients. Patient characteristics that may preclude MAC include obesity, significant gastroesophageal reflux disease, nausea, vomiting, and obstructive sleep apnea. General anesthesia is preferred over MAC for lead extractions because it provides a motionless patient for the cardiac electrophysiologist and increased control over patient hemodynamics and respiration in the event of a major vascular or cardiac complication. For high-risk lead extractions, sufficient intravascular access is key to patient safety. After induction of general anesthesia and intubation, a central line (such as a 9 Fr introducer sheath) is placed in the left femoral vein. A femoral venous central line is preferred because of the possible complication of a superior vena cava (SVC) tear, and the left side is selected to leave the right femoral vein for emergent cannulation for cardiopulmonary bypass. Large-bore central venous access is necessary for rapid volume resuscitation in the

event of acute bleeding and hemodynamic compromise and may be used for vasoactive infusions to support cardiac function in patients with limited reserve. A TEE probe is also placed and a comprehensive baseline examination is performed. In particular, the presence of lead thrombi/vegetations, pericardial or pleural effusions, and baseline amount of tricuspid regurgitation is assessed. In situations in which TEE is not available or the anesthesiologist is not trained in the use of TEE, intracardiac echocardiography (ICE) can be used by the cardiac electrophysiologist. ICE has been demonstrated to be both safe and efficacious for intraoperative procedural guidance and patient management.[22] Vasoactive infusions should be immediately available should the patient become hemodynamically unstable. After induction of anesthesia and satisfactory intravascular access, the patient should be prepped and draped in a fashion suitable to lead extraction as well as emergent sternotomy and femoral cannulation for cardiopulmonary bypass.[19–21]

Before the procedure, a time out is necessary to review the procedural plan and identify pertinent concerns of perioperative team members. The appropriate personnel should all be present for the time out and available at all times during the procedure. In addition to the cardiac electrophysiologist performing the procedure, the available team should include cardiac operating room nursing staff, a cardiothoracic surgeon, anesthesiologist, and perfusionist. Some institutions may choose to have a cardiac surgeon available on call, but not necessarily in the surgical suite during the procedure unless needed for urgent management of life-threatening complications. In such cases, the immediate availability of the cardiac

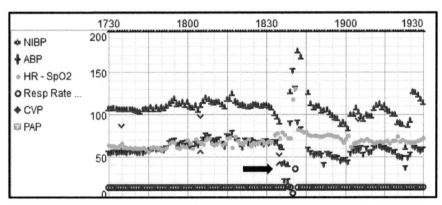

Fig. 5. Continuous hemodynamics from the anesthetic record of a patient undergoing extraction of leads that are 21 years old. The black arrow denotes a sudden drop in the invasive blood pressure measurement with simultaneously noted rapid collection of a large, circumferential pericardial effusion. Successful emergent sternotomy allowed the surgeon to identify a large laceration in the right atrium, which was quickly sutured shut and the bleeding was controlled. The patient made a full recovery with no neurologic sequelae.

surgeon should be confirmed during the time out. At this time, the cannulation strategy may also be reviewed in case of the need for emergent cardiopulmonary bypass. The heparin dose necessary for cardiopulmonary bypass should be discussed and the medication should be immediately available. All patients undergoing high-risk lead extraction need defibrillator and transcutaneous pacing pads placed before the procedure. In patients who are pacemaker dependent, a transvenous lead, implanted as described earlier, should be placed and connected to an external pacemaker generator. This provides the most reliable means of temporary pacing during and after the procedure. Once again, it should be confirmed that ICDs have had their tachyarrhythmia therapies disabled. Packed red blood cells must be present in the operating room or immediately available. In addition, cardiac surgical equipment should be present in the room. For some cases, a percutaneous pericardial drain and/or an SVC balloon may be of benefit if sternotomy and initiation of cardiopulmonary bypass is delayed or difficult, such as in patients with a history of prior sternotomy.[23] This may be of help when the cardiac surgeon is on-call but not scrubbed in to the procedure. Lastly, the time out should also include the patient's perioperative antibiotics and postoperative disposition for both an uncomplicated lead extraction and in the event of emergent sternotomy.[19–21]

Intraoperative TEE is valuable to perioperative management of patients undergoing high-risk lead extraction. Although many patients will have had a preoperative study, a comprehensive intraoperative baseline examination should be performed immediately before the procedure. In particular, the patient's biventricular function, valvular function, and device leads should be thoroughly assessed. Preexisting pericardial and pleural effusions should be assessed and quantified before the procedure to allow for early detection of bleeding in the perioperative setting. These pertinent findings confirmed during the baseline TEE should be discussed during the preprocedure time out so that all are aware of these findings should any changes occur during the procedure.

Continuous intraoperative TEE during lead extraction allows for early detection of intraoperative complications. In high-risk lead extractions, TEE is an invaluable tool in guiding clinical care. In a 2008 study by Endo and colleagues,[24] TEE provided clinically useful information in 16% of cases, including 5% that needed immediate surgical intervention. The mid-esophageal 4-chamber view and transgastric mid-papillary short axis view should be monitored frequently for evidence of any new or enlarging pericardial effusion. Communication between the cardiac electrophysiologist and anesthesiologist is important during key portions of the procedure to ensure rapid assessment of any clinical changes and a rapid response to potential complications. Any hemodynamic instability should be investigated with TEE.[24]

Intraoperative complications include SVC/right atrium rupture, tricuspid valve damage, RV rupture, RV inversion, pulmonary embolism and paradoxical embolism, and stroke.[25] Many of these complications can be rapidly and easily diagnosed with TEE. Tricuspid valve injury is suspected after worsened tricuspid regurgitation following removal of an RV lead. Pulmonary embolism or paradoxical embolism can be detected through the interval loss of previously visualized lead masses during the procedure. In extreme situations, the patient may develop an increased alveolar-arterial gradient, hypoxia, or decreased cerebral oxygen saturation. RV inversion may be detected on TEE during manual traction on the RV lead. If accompanied by significant hemodynamic instability the cardiac electrophysiologist should be alerted and release tension on the RV lead. Hemodynamics and echocardiographic images should be continuously assessed during key portions of the procedure to quickly identify complications. It should be noted, however, that some centers performing a high volume of lead extractions might choose not to use TEE routinely in all cases. Regoli and colleagues[26] found that TEE produced new findings during lead extraction in only 0.6% of cases, suggesting routine TEE for lead extraction may not be necessary. Even in situations when ICE is used in lieu of TEE or when no ECG guidance is used, TEE should be immediately available on site for the urgent assessment of hemodynamic instability.

Other measures may be used to help mitigate complications of lead extraction should they occur. If the patient has had prior cardiac surgery or chest radiation or if femoral cannulation may be difficult, a wire for an SVC balloon can be placed before lead extraction.[19] An SVC balloon can be placed and inflated in approximately 2 minutes and can mitigate bleeding until definitive control can be established. In addition, a pericardial drain can be placed to alleviate tamponade if sternotomy or initiation of cardiopulmonary bypass cannot be initiated expediently.[19,20]

After completion of the procedure, a comprehensive postoperative TEE examination should be completed to document any changes in valvular or ventricular function and to continue to monitor for the appearance of a new pericardial effusion. If any new complication is detected, the cardiac electrophysiologist, cardiac surgeon, and anesthesiologist should determine if an intervention is warranted and what new postoperative monitoring may be necessary.[24] The patient's hemodynamics and extent of the complication will help guide any necessary intervention.

POSTOPERATIVE CARE

In lead extractions without significant procedural or medical complications, patients can typically be extubated and monitored safely in the postanesthesia care unit (PACU). The procedure is usually well tolerated with only mild postoperative discomfort at the surgical site. In most cases, pain can be controlled through a combination of local anesthetic infiltration by the surgeon and nonopioid analgesic adjuncts. Patients should have continuous ECG and hemodynamic monitoring in the PACU. Postoperative changes in heart rate, rhythm, oxygenation, and/or hemodynamics warrant immediate further investigation. Given the potential for serious complications such as hemothorax, pneumothorax, and cardiac tamponade, the clinician should have a low threshold for use of transthoracic echocardiography or additional imaging in the expeditious diagnosis of significant hemodynamic changes.

Patients who experience major intraprocedural complications (vascular laceration, cardiac avulsion, cardiac arrest) requiring emergent surgical intervention should remain intubated and transferred to an ICU postoperatively. In addition, the anesthesiologist should consider ICU level care in those patients with significant cardiovascular comorbidities or those at highest risk of perioperative morbidity and mortality. A list of some of the comorbid conditions associated with complications or increased mortality can be found in **Table 2**. Patients requiring continuous intraoperative infusions of inotropes or vasoconstrictors that cannot be weaned at the end of the case should also be transferred to the ICU postoperatively for continued management and further diagnostic testing.

Postoperative care in a hospital unit with continuous ECG monitoring and experience in the management of temporary pacemakers and defibrillators will be necessary for many patients undergoing lead extraction. Patients with a history of malignant arrhythmias will need continuous monitoring of heart rhythm and immediate availability of defibrillation equipment if their ICD was not reimplanted (eg, due to device related infection). Similarly, pacemaker-dependent patients with a new temporary, externalized pacing system will need close postoperative monitoring because lead malfunction or lead dislodgement may lead to dangerous bradycardia, or even asystole.

Regardless of the postoperative disposition, the anesthesiologist should ensure that all of the following components of a safe and thorough transfer of care are discussed with the postoperative team:

- Original indication for device implantation
- Indication for explantation
- Arrhythmia history
- Pacemaker/ICD settings and underlying rhythm (if temporary or permanent device has been reimplanted)
- Comorbid medical conditions
- Intraoperative TEE findings
- Procedural complications
- Anesthetic complications
- Invasive lines and monitors
- Inotropic or vasoconstrictor infusions
- Planned or completed blood transfusion
- Relevant laboratory abnormalities
- Postoperative plan for anticoagulation if needed

As emphasized earlier, a multidisciplinary team-oriented approach with frequent and in-depth communication among all caregivers is critical in ensuring procedural success and good patient outcomes. The anesthesiologist's role as steward of patient safety must begin preoperatively and carry all the way through a safe transfer of care at the end of the case. The anesthesiologist should have a thorough understanding of CIED management, the surgical devices, and techniques used in lead extraction, procedural complications, and emergency equipment and techniques. Procedural complications must be identified quickly in order to save lives, and it is the prepared anesthesiologist, guided by appropriate invasive hemodynamic monitors and TEE, that is often the first to sound the alarm.

REFERENCES

1. Zhan C, Baine WB, Sedrakyan A, et al. Cardiac device implantation in the United States from 1997 through 2004: a population-based analysis. J Gen Intern Med 2008;23(1):13–9.
2. Voigt A, Shalaby A, Saba S. Continued rise in rates of cardiovascular implantable electronic device infections in the United States: temporal trends and causative insights. PacingClinElectrophysiol 2010; 33:414–9.
3. Wazni O, Epstein LM, Carrillo RG, et al. Lead extraction in the contemporary setting: the LExICon Study. JAm CollCardiol 2010;55(6):579–86.

4. Wilkoff BL, Love CJ, Byrd CL, et al. Transvenous lead extraction: heart Rhythm Society expert consensus on facilities, training, indications, and patient management. Heart Rhythm 2009;6(7): 1085–104.

5. Kusumoto FM, Schoenfeld MH, Wilkoff BL, et al. 2017 HRS expert consensus statement on cardiovascular implantable electronic device lead management and extraction. Heart Rhythm 2017; 14(12):e504–51.

6. Tarakji KG, Chan EJ, Cantillon DJ, et al. Cardiac implantable electronic device infections: presentation, management, and patient outcomes. Heart Rhythm 2010;7:1043–7.

7. Brunner MP, Changhong Y, Hussein AA, et al. Nomogram for predicting 30-day all-cause mortality after transvenous pacemaker and defibrillator lead extraction. Heart Rhythm 2015;12(12):2382–6.

8. Agarwal SK, Kamireddy S, Nemec J, et al. Predictors of complications of endovascular chronic lead extractions from pacemakers and defibrillators: a single-operator experience. J CardiovascElectrophysiol 2009;20:171–5.

9. Brunner MP, Cronin EM, Duarte VE, et al. Clinical predictors of adverse patient outcomes in an experience of more than 5,000 chronic endovascular pacemaker and defibrillator lead extractions. Heart Rhythm 2014;11(5):799–805.

10. Brunner MP, Cronin EM, Wazni O, et al. Outcomes of patients requiring emergent surgical or endovascular intervention for catastrophic complications during transvenous lead extraction. Heart Rhythm 2014;11(3):419–25.

11. Kay GN, Brinker JA, Kawanishi DT, et al. Risks of spontaneous injury and extraction of an active fixation pacemaker lead: report of the Accufix Multicenter Clinical Study and Worldwide Registry. Circulation 1999;100:2344–52.

12. Epstein LM, Love CJ, Wilkoff BL, et al. Superior vena cava defibrillators make transvenous lead extractions more challenging and riskier. J Am CollCardiol 2013;61:987–9.

13. Bernardes de Souza B, Benharash P, Esmalian F, et al. Value of a joint cardiac surgery—cardiac electrophysiology approach to lead extraction. J Card Surg 2015;30(11):874–6.

14. Bontempi L, Vassanelli F, Cerini M, et al. Predicting the difficulty of a lead extraction procedure: the LED index. J Cardiovasc Med 2014;15:668–73.

15. Bontempi L, Vassanelli F, Cerini M, et al. Predicting the difficulty of a transvenous lead extraction procedure: validation of the LED index. J CardiovascElectrophysiol 2017;28:811–8.

16. Pecha S, Aydin MA, Yildirim Y, et al. Transcutaneous lead implantation connected to an externalized pacemaker in patients with implantable cardiac defibrillator/pacemaker infection and pacemaker dependency. Europace 2013;15(8):1205–59.

17. Patel N, Azemi T, Zaeem F, et al. Vacuum assisted vegetation extraction for the management of large lead vegetations. J Card Surg 2013;28:321–4.

18. Nazmul MN, Cha YM, Lin G, et al. Percutaneous pacemaker or implantable cardioverter-defibrillator lead removal in an attempt to improve symptomatic tricuspid regurgitation. Europace 2013;15: 409–13.

19. Bhatia M, Safavi-Naeini P, Razavi M, et al. Anesthetic management of laser lead extraction for cardiovascular implantable electronic devices. SeminCardiothoracVascAnesth 2017;21(4):302–11.

20. Fermin L, Gebhard R, Azarrafiy R, et al. Pearls of wisdom for high-risk laser lead extractions: a focused review. AnesthAnalg 2017;10:1–7.

21. Maus TM, Shurter J, Nguyen L, et al. Multidisciplinary approach to transvenous lead extraction: a single center's experience. J CardiothoracVascAnesth 2015;29(2):265–70.

22. Bongiorni MG, Di Cori A, Soldati E, et al. Intracardiac echocardiography in patients with pacing and defibrillating leads: a feasibility study. Echocardiography 2008;25(6):632–8.

23. Azarrafiy R, Tsang DC, Boyle TA, et al. Compliant endovascular balloon reduces the lethality of superior vena cava tears during transvenous lead extractions. Heart Rhythm 2017;14(9):1400–4.

24. Endo Y, O'Mara JE, Weiner S, et al. Clinical utility of intraproceduraltransesophageal echocardiography during transvenous lead extraction. J Am SocEchocardiogr 2008;21(7):861–7.

25. Henrickson CA, Brinker JA. How to prevent, recognize and manage complications of lead extraction. Part III: procedural factors. Heart Rhythm 2008; 5(9):1352–4.

26. Regoli F, Caputo M, Conte G, et al. Clinical utility of routine use of continuous transesophageal echocardiography monitoring during transvenous lead extraction procedure. Heart Rhythm 2015;12(2): 313–20.

Lead Extraction Imaging

Pierce J. Vatterott, MD*, Imran S. Syed, MD, Akbar H. Khan, MD

KEYWORDS

- Lead extraction • Imaging • Cardiac CT • Echocardiography

KEY POINTS

- Imaging is an integral part of preprocedure planning for lead extraction.
- Procedural imaging is necessary for lead extraction.
- Lead binding sites are correlated with more complex extraction procedures.

INTRODUCTION

Lead implantation initiates a fibrous growth process that usually results in lead-vascular binding sites along the vascular path and electrode-myocardial interface.[1,2] Clinical factors are helpful in predicting fibrous adherences, but high individual patient variance exists.[2–4] Significant adhesions and perforation of vascular and cardiac tissue affect the difficulty and risks of lead extraction.[3] Removal of adhered or perforated leads can result in significant complications, such as superior vena cava (SVC) tear, cardiac avulsion, and even death.[3,4]

Imaging is critical in defining potential vascular adhesions, cardiac perforations and any aberrant lead course, and modifying the approach to the specific challenges of the case.[3,4] Several imaging modalities assist the extractor, from a simple chest radiograph (CXR) to computed tomography (CT) imaging. A successful lead extraction program requires close collaboration between the cardiologist/cardiac EP, cardiac surgeon, and imaging colleagues.

Lead extraction requires both preprocedural and procedural imaging (**Box 1**). Preprocedural imaging allows for early identification of procedural challenges. This information often modifies procedural strategies and may impact the decision to extract.

PREPROCEDURAL CHEST RADIOGRAPH

A posterior-anterior (PA) and lateral CXR is a simple and widely available tool that contains a wealth of information (**Box 2**).[5,6] Early review of the CXR is essential and can aid in directing other preprocedural imaging. The CXR may demonstrate inaccuracies in reported lead information, such as the number and location of the leads. The presence of sternal wires and evidence of prior coronary artery bypass graft surgery (CABG) should remind the CT reader to define graft locations in case of urgent sternotomy. The following cases are examples of crucial information provided by the CXR.

Fig. 1 shows a CXR of a 60-year-old man with dilated cardiomyopathy (ejection fraction [EF] 25%), complete heart block, and atrial fibrillation referred for extraction and upgrade to a biventricular implantable cardioverter defibrillator (ICD). Two abandoned unipolar right-sided leads (implanted 16 years before) are visualized, with the right ventricular (RV) lead severed. The atrial lead is an extendable retractable lead, and the RV unipolar lead is passive. A left-sided single

Statement of disclosure: Dr P.J. Vatterott receives consulting fees from Phillips Medical, Medtronic, and Inspire and teaching support from Cook Medical. Dr A.H. Khan and Dr I.S. Syed do not report any commercial or financial conflicts of interest. This work was published without any funding support.
United Heart & Vascular Clinic, Allina Health System, 225 North Smith Avenue, Suite 400, St Paul, MN 55102, USA
* Corresponding author.
E-mail address: pierce.vatterott@allina.com

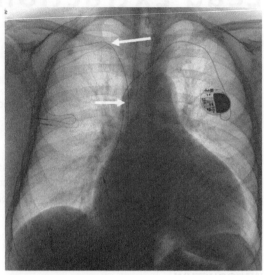

Fig. 1. PA CXR from a 60-year-old man referred for extraction and upgrade to a biventricular ICD. Arrows point to the severed proximal and distal ends of one of the right-sided pacing leads.

Box 1
Preprocedural and procedural imaging tests

Preprocedural

Chest radiograph (CXR)

Echocardiogram

Computed tomography (CT) scan

Subclavian venogram

Procedural

Subclavian venogram

Cine imaging fluoroscopy

SVC angiography

Transesophageal echocardiography (TEE)

Intracardiac echocardiography (ICE)

---

pacemaker generator is connected to a bipolar extendable retractable lead (implanted 5 years before) with the tip in the RV apex. Identification of the cut and retracted RV lead allowed early

---

Box 2
Checklist for reviewing chest radiograph before lead extraction

Passive, fixed screw or extendable/retractable leads

Unusual lead requiring special extraction technique (ie, Medtronic LV Starfix lead)

Any unaccounted for leads

Abandoned leads

Damaged leads

Prior approach for implantation

    Subclavian/axillary/cephalic access

    Tunneled leads

    Medial access with possible clavicular crush injury

    Epicardial leads. Is the exit site from the thorax remote from pocket?

Unusual lead loop or course

Pacing or ICD leads

Dual coil or single coil ICD lead

SVC coil location

Evidence of extruded cables

Twiddler syndrome

Inadequate connector pin seating

Perforation of heart or vascular system

Unusual cardiac anatomy

---

development of an appropriate extraction strategy. An anticipation of an upgrade to the previous left-sided device warrants establishment of venous patency.

Figs. 2 and **3** show a CXR of a pacemaker-dependent man with presyncopal spells, prior CABG, EF 40%, and chronic atrial fibrillation. Device interrogation during left arm movement demonstrated ventricular electrogram noise with pacing inhibition.

Initial CXR (see **Fig. 2**A) shows a dual-chamber pacemaker system. Digital magnification (see **Fig. 2**B) highlights clavicular lead crush. These leads may be adhered near the clavicle, requiring direct surgical access or an extraction cutting tool for removal.

Reviewing the lateral CXR is critical (see **Fig. 2**C).[6] Here the ventricular lead courses to an atypical posterior cardiac location demonstrated by echocardiography to be the left ventricle (LV). A decision to not extract was made. For comparison, a postprocedure CXR is shown (see **Fig. 2**D) delineating the additional RV and LV leads.

Extraction of dual coil ICD leads is associated with a higher incidence of vascular tears.[7,8] ICD coils increase vascular binding sites.[7,8] Preprocedure, the physician should note lead course, coil location, and potential vascular binding sites (see **Fig. 3**A). CXR illustrates an SVC coil that courses from the left innominate to the superior SVC (see **Fig. 3**B). The

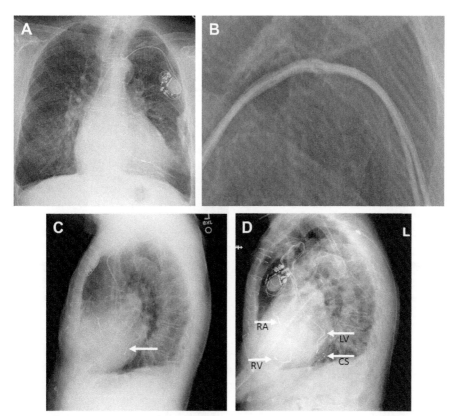

Fig. 2. (*A*) PA CXR from an 89-year-old pacemaker-dependent man referred for lightheaded spells and pacemaker failure to pace. (*B*) Magnification of the leads at the clavicle demonstrates lead disruption with probable crush injury. (*C*) Lateral CXR from the same patient illustrates a ventricular pacing lead coursing to an atypical posterior location in the cardiac silhouette. (*D*) Same patient postprocedure lateral CXR. Arrows illustrate new right ventricle and coronary sinus pacing leads, old RA, and LV leads.

associated lateral CXR delineates the typical innominate posterior course (see **Fig. 3**C). CXR characterizes an SVC coil that extends from the superior SVC to the right atrium (RA) junction. Review of Cleveland Clinic cases suggests most SVC tears occur at that SVC-RA junction[7] (see **Fig. 3**D). CXR illustrates 2 potentially entangled ICD leads with multiple possible vasculature and lead to lead binding sites. During extraction, traction on one lead may affect the other lead and its vascular binding sites.

Subclavian Venogram

A subclavian venogram can be obtained preprocedure, during the procedure, or can be accomplished with the preprocedure CT scan. Partial occlusion with leads outside the contrast lumen illustrates subclavian and innominate vasculature binding sites.[9,10] Total vessel occlusion requires planning for any implantation of new leads after extraction.

PREPROCEDURAL COMPUTED TOMOGRAPHIC SCAN

Cardiac CT has an important role in preprocedural planning. Contrast-enhanced electrocardiographic (ECG)-gated multidetector CT allows for assessment of vascular patency and lead binding sites, lead positions, and most importantly, evidence of perforation. In fact, cardiac CT has been proposed as the gold standard technique for assessment of lead position and perforation. The main issue with cardiac CT involves artifacts that can hinder accurate identification of lead tip location, but this can be reduced with modern techniques.

Assessment of Device Lead Position in the Right Atrium and Right Ventricle

Identification of lead tip position in the RV can help assess the risk of complications such as perforation. The risk is present with nonseptal lead location and highest with apical insertion

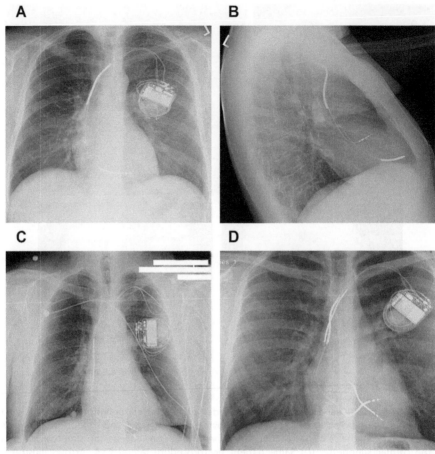

Fig. 3. (*A*) PA CXR illustrating an SVC coil that extends from the innominate to the superior portion of the SVC. (*B*) A lateral CXR from the same patient illustrating the typical posterior lead path from innominate to SVC. (*C*) PA CXR characterizing an SVC coil extends the length of the SVC to the SVC right atrial junction. (*D*) PA CXR illustrating 2 ICD leads potentially entangled in the SVC.

where the RV wall is thinnest. Cardiac CT is ideal for assessing lead position in the geometrically complex RV and is superior to other modalities.[11] Multiple studies have demonstrated that CXR and fluoroscopy are inaccurate in distinguishing septal from nonseptal insertion, with only 21% to 56% concordance with CT.[11,12] In particular, leads demonstrated by CT to be on the anterior free wall are often misidentified on CXR and fluoroscopy as being septal. **Fig. 4** illustrates the

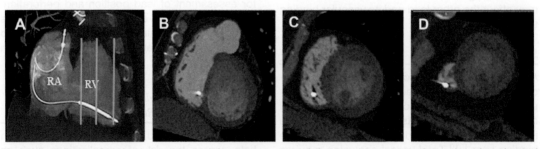

Fig. 4. Assessment of RV lead tip position. (*A*) Long-axis view of the RV is reconstructed. Basal, mid, and apical slices are obtained (*blue lines*). (*B*) Basal RV short axis. (*C*) Mid RV short axis. (*D*) RV lead tip is seen to terminate in the RV apex in the RV apical inferior segment.

segmentation technique for identifying lead tip position in the RV. RA leads and LV leads can also be reliably identified using a multiplanar technique.

Assessment of Lead Perforation in the Right Atrium and Right Ventricle

Preprocedure cardiac CT can identify unrecognized cardiac perforation. Late lead perforation (>1 month after implantation) is rare. Preprocedural identification of lead perforation may impact the decision to extract as well as the extraction technique. The primary challenge with identifying lead perforation relates to metal and motion artifacts. A dedicated lead extraction CT scanning protocol helps to minimize artifacts and produce high-quality images (**Figs. 5** and **6**). Motion artifact is reduced with ECG-gating, typically with diastolic acquisition. Metal "blooming" artifact can be reduced by postprocessing algorithms with appropriate windowing and "sharp" kernels, whereas metal streak artifacts can be reduced with multiplanar image reformatting.

Early studies using non-ECG-gated and non-contrast CT for determination of lead perforation reported relatively high rates of "occult" lead perforation that were likely overestimates due to suboptimal image quality.[13,14] Recent studies have used ECG-gated contrast-enhanced cardiac CT, which increases accuracy.[15,16] In the study by Lewis and colleagues,[15] one of 30 patients (3%) had significant RV lead perforation with lead tip 1 cm beyond the epicardium. In the study by Pang and colleagues,[16] 2 of 52 patients (4%) had clinically significant RV lead perforation with leads tips between 5 and 15 mm beyond the epicardium with pericardial effusion, and no patient had RA lead perforation. The clinical significance of isolated radiologic "perforations" without pericardial effusion or changes in pacing parameters remains uncertain. At the authors' institution, they routinely report RV lead insertion site (septal, free wall, apical cap) and degree of penetration. High-risk features are evidence of RV lead perforation or any lead tip in the true RV apex.

RA lead perforations are rare. RA leads are typically positioned in the appendage, which is trabeculated and thicker than the remainder of the RA. An autopsy study demonstrated active fixation RA leads typically exhibit superficial penetration into the endocardium compared with RV leads.[17] Although RA tenting is sometimes noted and considered by some extractors to be a high-risk feature, in clinical practice, many of these leads can be safely removed without complications.[15]

Assessment of Central Venous Structures and Vascular Adherence

Knowledge of SVC and axillary/subclavian vein patency and presence of any stenosis are desirable. Vascular adherence or extraluminal lead location, especially near the SVC-atrial junction, is a high-risk feature. A dedicated CT protocol with imaging from the neck through the heart with contrast injection in the arm, ipsilateral to the device, allows for comprehensive assessment of venous patency, thrombosis, and vascular

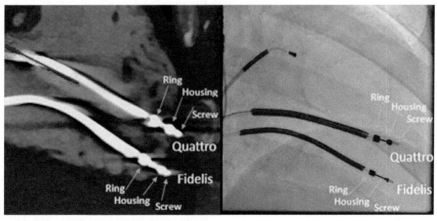

Fig. 5. High-resolution imaging of device leads can be obtained with a dedicated lead extraction cardiac CT protocol. Multi-planar reformatted long-axis view of the right ventricle in a patient with Sprint Quattro and Fidelis leads. Beam hardening artifact is present but does not interfere with diagnostic interpretability. Familiarity with device lead components is helpful for accurate image interpretation. (*Courtesy of* Medtronic, Inc, Minneapolis, MN. © Medtronic 2018.)

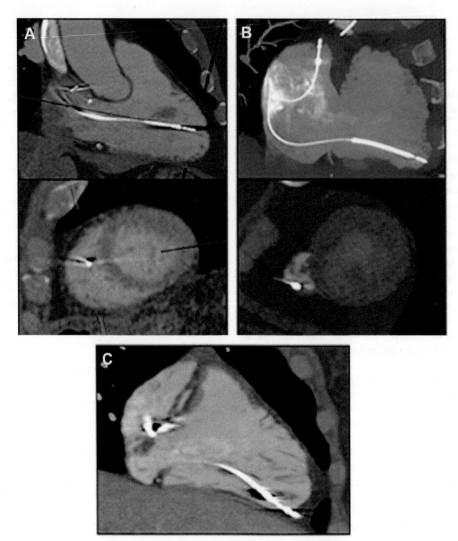

Fig. 6. Assessment of RV lead tip penetration into the RV myocardium. (*A*) Top panel demonstrates long-axis RV view and bottom panel demonstrates short-axis view. Device lead tip is inserted in to an RV trabeculation. (*B*) Top panel demonstrates long-axis RV view and bottom panel demonstrates short-axis view. Device lead tip is inserted in to the RV apical inferior segment myocardium without evidence of perforation. (*C*) Example of RV lead tip radiologic perforation. Lead tip extends beyond the RV epicardium. No evidence of pericardial effusion.

adherence. In one study, CT assessment of vascular adherence was associated with longer laser times and larger sheath sizes.[15] Virtual CT-intravascular ultrasound (IVUS) can be performed with cross-sectional analysis of the SVC lumen in manner similar to intracardiac echocardiography (ICE) (**Fig. 7**).

Summary

Preprocedural cardiac CT allows for assessment of lead position and lead perforation in the cardiac chambers as well as important adjunctive information such as venous patency and thrombosis, and

vascular adherence. Large multicenter trials are needed to establish if preprocedural CT ultimately reduces complications.

PREPROCEDURAL ECHOCARDIOGRAPHY

Echocardiography provides comprehensive structural and functional assessment of the heart and is important in the preprocedural evaluation of patients undergoing lead extraction. Indeed, it may be findings consistent with endocarditis or lead-related severe tricuspid regurgitation on a transthoracic echocardiogram (TTE) that prompts initial evaluation for lead extraction.

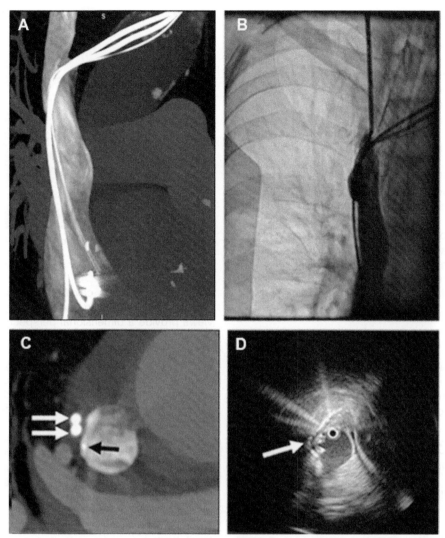

Fig. 7. Example of vascular adherence of 2 device leads into the SVC wall. (*A*) CT venogram demonstrating long-axis view of SVC with 2 device leads outside the contrast lumen. (*B*) SVC venography confirms CT findings. (*C*) CT-virtual IVUS demonstrates that both device leads are outside the contrast lumen. (*D*) ICE at the same location delineates considerable scar on the lead. Although the lead is outside the contrast lumen, it remains within the structural SVC lumen.

Once the need for lead extraction has been established, the TTE can provide baseline assessment of cardiac chamber function, valve pathology, and pericardial effusion. TTE can also confirm or diagnose lead malposition, such as inadvertent LV lead placement.[18]

When device infection is suspected, it is important to obtain detailed information regarding the presence or absence of vegetations on the valves and leads, impact on valve function, and vegetation characteristics, such as size and mobility. Previously, patients with vegetations (>1 cm) were treated with surgery due to concerns regarding the potential for septic embolization. However,

recent data have shown that even patients with larger vegetations (up to 3 or 4 cm) can safely undergo standard percutaneous lead extraction techniques.[19,20]

The tricuspid valve needs to be evaluated for the presence and severity of regurgitation. Device leads are increasingly recognized as a cause of significant tricuspid regurgitation.[21] Impingement of the valve leaflets, adherence to the leaflets, leaflet perforation, lead entanglement within the chordal apparatus, and mal-coaptation related to multiple leads have been described as potential mechanisms and can be evaluated with TTE.[22,23] Importantly, lead-related tricuspid regurgitation is independently associated with increased morbidity and mortality.[24] Conversely, tricuspid regurgitation is a known complication of transcutaneous lead extraction.[25] This further underscores the importance of preprocedure assessment of tricuspid valve function. Recently, 3-dimensional echocardiography has been shown to be of increasing utility in describing the spatial relationship between the tricuspid valve leaflets and the device leads as well as severity of the associated tricuspid regurgitation.[24,25]

Although the specificity of TTE for detecting valvular and lead vegetations is high (>98%), a lower sensitivity of 75% does not allow for reliable exclusion of vegetations. The higher sensitivity (>90%) of transesophageal echocardiography (TEE) makes it the imaging modality of choice for evaluation of endocarditis, especially when TTE images are suboptimal or when the suspicion for endocarditis is high despite an unremarkable TTE.[26]

PROCEDURAL IMAGING

Procedural imaging has 2 purposes: to further exploration of any concerns suggested by preprocedural imaging and to monitor the patient during the procedure.

Fluoroscopic Imaging

High-quality fluoroscopic imaging is required for the lead extraction procedure.[4] Issues delineated include lead to lead binding, unusual lead

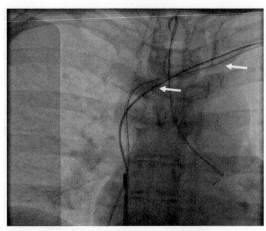

Fig. 9. White arrows delineating calcified scar in this cine still frame.

paths or tip locations, calcified scar tissue along the lead, and defining lead integrity. Angled views provide a dimensional perspective. **Fig. 8** illustrates a redundant lead loop in the right innominate. Extraction challenges include inability to pass a locking stylet and right innominate vascular binding sites. **Fig. 9** delineates calcified scar along the lead bodies and between the leads. A cutting tool–powered sheath was required for removal.

In the presence of lead to lead binding, it is essential to understand that manipulation of one lead affects attached leads. High-quality fluoroscopic imaging is essential in delineating lead integrity issues, such as lead fracture, insulation disruption, and presence and extent of cable externalization in compromised Riata and Biotronik leads.[4,27]

Echocardiography

The use of TEE during extraction is routine at many centers. It allows rapid intraprocedural complication assessment for pericardial effusion, tamponade, acute valve disruption, pulmonary embolism, and vascular injury.[28,29] Other centers use ICE. TTE is not used because of the limited imaging windows available during the procedure.

The information provided by ICE is additive to other imaging modalities especially in its definition of vascular binding sites.[30,31] The presence of vascular binding sites is associated with more complex procedures and higher procedural complications.[30,31] Phased-array ICE is the dominant modality used during electrophysiological procedures.[30] The authors' laboratory has used rotational ICE during extraction for more

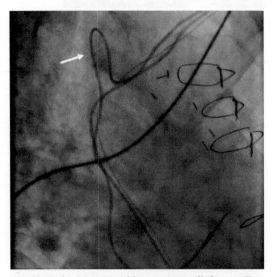

Fig. 8. Right anterior oblique cine still frame illustrating a redundant lead loop within the right innominate.

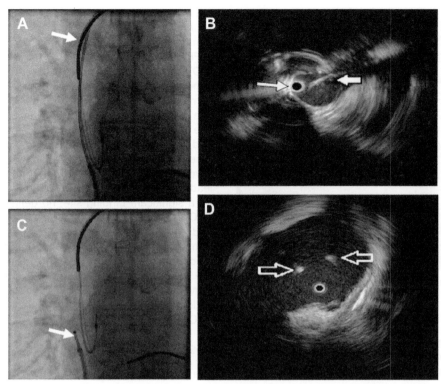

Fig. 10. (A) Fluoroscopic image of ICE catheter imaging position. (B) Corresponding ICE to panel (A) illustrating leads within the left innominate vein as it enters the SVC. (C) Fluoroscopic image of the ICE catheter imaging position, panel (D) corresponding ICE to panel (C) illustrating leads position within the RA.

than 20 years, which provides a high-resolution near-field image.

The ICE catheter and deflectable sheath are advanced to the right innominate and then gradually pulled down to the RA evaluating possible any lead vascular binding sites. **Fig. 10** delineates the range of area examined by ICE. Areas of concern are documented on both ICE and fluoroscopy allowing possible reexamination during the procedure. **Fig. 11** illustrates pacing leads within the SVC lumen and no vascular binding sites. In comparison, **Fig. 12** illustrates a lead with SVC vascular binding.

After SVC scanning, the ICE catheter is positioned within the RA for pericardial space

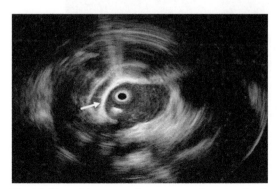

Fig. 11. The white arrow demonstrates 2 pacing leads adhered to each other but no vascular binding.

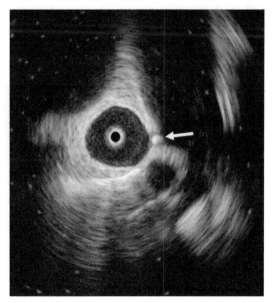

Fig. 12. The white arrow illustrates the SVC lead vascular binding site.

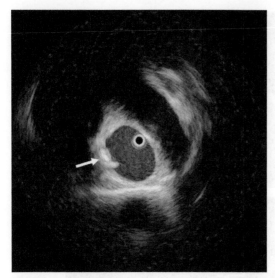

Fig. 13. An ICD lead and pacing lead adhered to the SVC wall.

monitoring. However, the benefits of continuous echocardiographic procedural monitoring have been questioned.[29]

COMPUTED TOMOGRAPHIC SCAN AND INTRACARDIAC ECHOCARDIOGRAPHY CORRELATIONS

ICE can be used to study SVC areas of concern when the preprocedural CT scan illustrates leads outside the SVC contrast lumen. In the authors' experience, CT scans and ICE typically correlate well in demonstrating lead position within the lumen but differ in delineating vascular binding sites. Contrast studies appear to be limited by

how contrast flows, whereas ICE provides local tissue characteristics. **Fig. 7** is such a demonstration.

Fig. 7A–C illustrate that 2 of the 3 leads (one ICD and one pacing) are outside of the contrast lumen. ICE image (see **Fig. 7**D) taken at the same SVC level does show considerable scar tissue on the leads, but no SVC vascular binding site. The SVC wall is still visible as independent and not contiguous with the leads. During real-time imaging, the leads and SVC moved independently. A comparison ICE image (**Fig. 13**) shows leads demonstrated at open heart procedure to be a significant binding site; no definition of the SVC wall is seen. During real-time imaging, leads and wall moved in synchrony. **Fig. 14** images are from a patient with a significant lead vascular binding site. ICE image (see **Fig. 14**A) delineates the vascular binding site. After ICE monitored removal with a powered cutting tool (Spectranetics Tight Rail), **Fig. 14**B illustrates the residual SVC scar.

POSTPROCEDURAL IMAGING

The postprocedure echocardiogram can be used to assess for pericardial effusions and evaluation of the tricuspid valve for regurgitation. New or worsening tricuspid regurgitation is a known complication of lead extraction and reported to be more frequent with use of laser sheaths. Photochemical destruction, motor force, and mechanical damage from the outer sheath have been postulated as possible mechanisms for tricuspid valve injury.[32] It is still unclear if extraction of the RV lead in this setting will improve the degree of tricuspid regurgitation or outcome.[21,33]

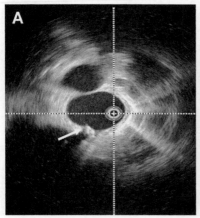
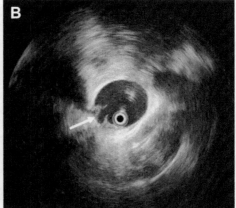

Fig. 14. (A) ICD and pacing leads are adhered to the wall of the SVC before extraction. (B) The white arrow shows where scar is remaining in the vessel after the leads have been extracted.

SUMMARY

Imaging is a critical part of the lead extraction process. By integrating the information gained through preprocedure and procedural imaging, the physician is able to better manage the challenges of lead extraction for each individual patient.

ACKNOWLEDGMENTS

The acknowledge Ryan Gage's assistance in the preparation of this article for publication.

REFERENCES

1. Epstein AE, Kay GN, Plumb VJ, et al. Gross and microscopic pathological changes associated with nonthoracotomy implantable defibrillator leads. Circulation 1998;98(15):1517–24.

2. Segreti L, Di Cori A, Soldati E, et al. Major predictors of fibrous adherences in transvenous implantable cardioverter-defibrillator lead extraction. Heart Rhythm 2014;11(12):2196–201.

3. Kennergren C, Bjurman C, Wiklund R, et al. A single-centre experience of over one thousand lead extractions. Europace 2009;11(5):612–7.

4. Kusumoto FM, Schoenfeld MH, Wilkoff BL, et al. 2017 HRS expert consensus statement on cardiovascular implantable electronic device lead management and extraction. Heart Rhythm 2017; 14(12):e503–51.

5. Burney K, Burchard F, Papouchado M, et al. Cardiac pacing systems and implantable cardiac defibrillators (ICDs): a radiological perspective of equipment, anatomy and complications. Clin Radiol 2004;59(8): 699–708.

6. Furman S. Chest PA and lateral. Pacing Clin Electrophysiol 1993;16(5 Pt 1):953.

7. Brunner MP, Cronin EM, Wazni O, et al. Outcomes of patients requiring emergent surgical or endovascular intervention for catastrophic complications during transvenous lead extraction. Heart Rhythm 2014;11(3):419–25.

8. Epstein LM, Love CJ, Wilkoff BL, et al. Superior vena cava defibrillator coils make transvenous lead extraction more challenging and riskier. J Am Coll Cardiol 2013;61(9):987–9.

9. Abu-El-Haija B, Bhave PD, Campbell DN, et al. Venous stenosis after transvenous lead placement: a study of outcomes and risk factors in 212 consecutive patients. J Am Heart Assoc 2015;4(8): e001878.

10. Li X, Ze F, Wang L, et al. Prevalence of venous occlusion in patients referred for lead extraction: implications for tool selection. Europace 2014;16(12):1795–9.

11. Moore P, Coucher J, Ngai S, et al. Imaging and right ventricular pacing lead position: a comparison of CT, MRI, and echocardiography. Pacing Clin Electrophysiol 2016;39(4):382–92.

12. Pang BJ, Joshi SB, Lui EH, et al. Validation of conventional fluoroscopic and ECG criteria for right ventricular pacemaker lead position using cardiac computed tomography. Pacing Clin Electrophysiol 2014;37(4):495–504.

13. Balabanoff C, Gaffney CE, Ghersin E, et al. Radiographic and electrocardiography-gated noncontrast cardiac CT assessment of lead perforation: modality comparison and interobserver agreement. J Cardiovasc Comput Tomogr 2014;8(5):384–90.

14. Hirschl DA, Jain VR, Spindola-Franco H, et al. Prevalence and characterization of asymptomatic pacemaker and ICD lead perforation on CT. Pacing Clin Electrophysiol 2007;30(1):28–32.

15. Lewis RK, Pokorney SD, Greenfield RA, et al. Preprocedural ECG-gated computed tomography for prevention of complications during lead extraction. Pacing Clin Electrophysiol 2014;37(10): 1297–305.

16. Pang BJ, Lui EH, Joshi SB, et al. Pacing and implantable cardioverter defibrillator lead perforation as assessed by multiplanar reformatted ECG-gated cardiac computed tomography and clinical correlates. Pacing Clin Electrophysiol 2014;37(5): 537–45.

17. Dvorak P, Novak M, Kamaryt P, et al. Histological findings around electrodes in pacemaker and implantable cardioverter-defibrillator patients: comparison of steroid-eluting and non-steroid-eluting electrodes. Europace 2012;14(1):117–23.

18. Van Gelder BM, Bracke FA, Oto A, et al. Diagnosis and management of inadvertently placed pacing and ICD leads in the left ventricle: a multicenter experience and review of the literature. Pacing Clin Electrophysiol 2000;23(5):877–83.

19. Grammes JA, Schulze CM, Al-Bataineh M, et al. Percutaneous pacemaker and implantable cardioverter-defibrillator lead extraction in 100 patients with intracardiac vegetations defined by transesophageal echocardiogram. J Am Coll Cardiol 2010;55(9):886–94.

20. Meier-Ewert HK, Gray ME, John RM. Endocardial pacemaker or defibrillator leads with infected vegetations: a single-center experience and consequences of transvenous extraction. Am Heart J 2003;146(2):339–44.

21. Lin G, Nishimura RA, Connolly HM, et al. Severe symptomatic tricuspid valve regurgitation due to permanent pacemaker or implantable cardioverter-defibrillator leads. J Am Coll Cardiol 2005;45(10): 1672–5.

22. Mediratta A, Addetia K, Yamat M, et al. 3D echocardiographic location of implantable device leads and mechanism of associated tricuspid regurgitation. JACC Cardiovasc Imaging 2014;7(4):337–47.

23. Seo Y, Ishizu T, Nakajima H, et al. Clinical utility of 3-dimensional echocardiography in the evaluation of tricuspid regurgitation caused by pacemaker leads. Circ J 2008;72(9):1465–70.

24. Hoke U, Auger D, Thijssen J, et al. Significant lead-induced tricuspid regurgitation is associated with poor prognosis at long-term follow-up. Heart 2014; 100(12):960–8.

25. Coffey JO, Sager SJ, Gangireddy S, et al. The impact of transvenous lead extraction on tricuspid valve function. Pacing Clin Electrophysiol 2014; 37(1):19–24.

26. De Castro S, Cartoni D, d'Amati G, et al. Diagnostic accuracy of transthoracic and multiplane transesophageal echocardiography for valvular perforation in acute infective endocarditis: correlation with anatomic findings. Clin Infect Dis 2000; 30(5):825–6.

27. Liu J, Rattan R, Adelstein E, et al. Fluoroscopic screening of asymptomatic patients implanted with the recalled Riata lead family. Circ Arrhythm Electrophysiol 2012;5(4):809–14.

28. Hilberath JN, Burrage PS, Shernan SK, et al. Rescue transoesophageal echocardiography for refractory haemodynamic instability during transvenous lead extraction. Eur Heart J Cardiovasc Imaging 2014; 15(8):926–32.

29. Regoli F, Caputo M, Conte G, et al. Clinical utility of routine use of continuous transesophageal echocardiography monitoring during transvenous lead extraction procedure. Heart Rhythm 2015;12(2): 313–20.

30. Sadek MM, Cooper JM, Frankel DS, et al. Utility of intracardiac echocardiography during transvenous lead extraction. Heart Rhythm 2017;14(12):1779–85.

31. Yakish SJ, Narula A, Foley R, et al. Superior vena cava echocardiography as a screening tool to predict cardiovascular implantable electronic device lead fibrosis. J Cardiovasc Ultrasound 2015;23(1): 27–31.

32. Roeffel S, Bracke F, Meijer A, et al. Transesophageal echocardiographic evaluation of tricuspid valve regurgitation during pacemaker and implantable cardioverter defibrillator lead extraction. Pacing Clin Electrophysiol 2002;25(11):1583–6.

33. Nazmul MN, Cha YM, Lin G, et al. Percutaneous pacemaker or implantable cardioverter-defibrillator lead removal in an attempt to improve symptomatic tricuspid regurgitation. Europace 2013;15(3): 409–13.

A Practical Approach to Lead Removal
Transvenous Tools and Techniques

Felix Krainski, MD*, Victor Pretorius, MBChB,
Ulrika Birgersdotter-Green, MD

KEYWORDS

- Cardiac implantable electronic devices • Lead extraction • Lead management

KEY POINTS

- Transvenous lead removal is a complex skillset requiring knowledge of all available tools and vascular access techniques to produce successful outcomes.
- Optimal tool selection varies based on the lead-tissue interface, fibrotic lesion characteristics, patient characteristics aspects, lead properties, lead dwell time, and operator experience.
- Superior implant vein and femoral vein access are the most common approaches to lead removal for which the current state-of-the-art tools and techniques are presented in this article.

INTRODUCTION

Removal of cardiovascular implantable electronic device (CIED) leads is of paramount importance in the management of patients presenting with CIED infections, need for device upgrades, and lead failure in an environment of ever-expanding device placement indications, increasing patient longevity and changing lead design and technology.[1] Growing numbers of physicians are expanding their skillset to include extraction procedures, a generally safe yet potentially high-risk treatment. As such, mastering the skill of lead extraction is essential to establish and maintain safe and effective patient care. The 2009 Heart Rhythm Society (HRS) Transvenous Lead Extraction Consensus on Facilities, Training, Indications, and Patient Management document and 2017 HRS Consensus Statement on CIED Lead Management and Extraction are excellent resources for every aspect a comprehensive lead management program should encompass.[2,3] This article will serve as a practical resource presenting essential tools and vascular approaches of transvenous lead extraction.

HISTORICAL PERSPECTIVE

The field of lead extraction first arose through the necessity of completely removing infected CIED systems and soon included preventive or anticipatory lead removal indications to avoid venous obstruction, lead-lead interactions, and other lead-related complications when lead abandonment does not appear favorable.[1] In concert with technological advances, transvenous lead removal techniques have evolved from direct traction and weight and pulley ("Buck traction") (**Fig. 1**) to include mechanical and laser sheaths, progressive dissection, countertraction, and grasping and snaring instruments using various vascular sites, including access via mainly a superior approach from the implant vein, and also an inferior approach from the femoral vein.[4] In some cases,

Disclosures: None.
University of California San Diego Medical Center, La Jolla, CA, USA
* Corresponding author. Department of Cardiac Electrophysiology, 9453 Medical Center Drive, MC 7411, La Jolla, CA 92037.
E-mail address: fkrainski@ucsd.edu

Card Electrophysiol Clin 10 (2018) 637–650
https://doi.org/10.1016/j.ccep.2018.08.002

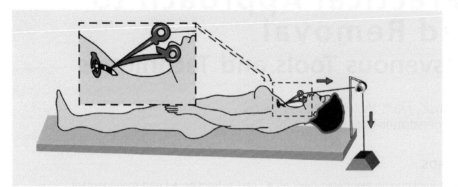

Fig. 1. Lead removal using weight and pulley, also called Buck traction. (*From* Diemberger I, Mazzotti A, Giulia MB, et al. From lead management to implanted patient management: systematic review and meta-analysis of the last 15 years of experience in lead extraction. Expert Rev Med Devices 2013;10(4):553; with permission.)

additional internal jugular vein access can be helpful.[5] Tools have been either specifically designed for lead extraction in the case of a superior approach from the implant vein (laser and mechanical extraction sheaths) or, in the case of femoral approach, adopted from procedures used to grasp tissue samples and retrieve wires, catheters, and other foreign bodies from the central circulation.[6]

DEFINITIONS

The 2009 and 2017 HRS lead management statements define the process of lead removal as (1) lead explant when no additional tools apart from implant stylets are used and when lead dwell time is <1 year, and (2) lead extraction when specialized tools not typically used during implant are required or when lead dwell time is >1 year. The same documents define the procedural outcome as (1) complete procedural success, when all targeted leads can be removed from the vascular space in their entirety; (2) clinical success, when all targeted leads can be removed or when a small portion of the lead (<4 cm) is retained that does not negatively impact the outcome goals of the procedure; and (3) failure, when complete procedural or clinical success cannot be achieved, or when the procedure results in development of any permanently disabling complication or procedure-related death.[2,3]

BASIC CONSIDERATIONS

The necessity of approaching leads via various vascular access sites is a result of the variability of clinical scenarios demanding high operator flexibility in switching from one mode of access to another and ability to use full range of available tools. Notably, the operator should have access to all available extraction tools and cardiovascular

approaches to manage unexpected lead behavior and prevent or temporize complications.[2] Although superior venous access via the implant vein is generally the primary approach for lead removal, snaring leads through femoral venous access or a combination of both often becomes necessary for removal of cut leads or lead fragments attached to or free-floating in the venous system, heart, or pulmonary arteries and in the case of femoral or external iliac venous lead implantation.[1,6] Although some centers prefer a strictly femoral access approach with data suggesting safety and efficacy equivalent to other approaches, fluoroscopy and procedure times are longer.[7] Importantly, the ELECTRa European registry found that extraction procedures that used femoral access were actually associated with a higher complication rate.[8] Nevertheless, femoral snaring is often used as a bail-out for incomplete failed extraction from above. Optimal tool selection varies based on the lead-tissue interface, fibrotic lesion characteristics, patient characteristics aspects, lead properties, lead dwell time, and operator experience.[2] Regardless of the site of access, extractions are best performed under general anesthesia, with chest and abdomen prepared for emergency sternotomy and/or laparotomy. Continuous intraoperative transesophageal or potentially intracardiac echocardiography is recommended for timely identification of complications. Arterial access is essential for hemodynamic monitoring and central venous access for administration of medications, blood products and, depending on the risk assessment, femoral venous access for placement of contingency equipment such as a superior vena cava (SVC) wire and rescue balloon system. Furthermore, lead removal procedures should always be a multidisciplinary effort among cardiac electrophysiologists, cardiothoracic surgeons, anesthesia, infectious disease specialists, nursing, and technologists.[1]

SUPERIOR (IMPLANT VEIN) APPROACH

Superior access via the implant vein is now generally considered the primary approach for lead extractions. Over the past 2 decades, various tools have been developed and refined specifically for extraction purposes via the lead vein. The superior approach is advantageous in most clinical scenarios:

- Complete or partial extraction of CIED systems. After opening the device pocket, targeted leads can be selected and extracted individually. Generally, lead integrity of retained leads remains preserved.
- In patients requiring reimplantation of a new CIED system or new leads, the sheaths used for extraction serve as a venous access conduit even in previously occluded or heavily fibrotic venous systems.
- As opposed to most femoral extractions, the superior approach generally allows for placement of locking stylets providing the necessary mechanical tensile strength to successfully extract the lead and prevent disintegration.
- Superior venous access can be combined with a femoral approach in challenging situations.

Technique

Several steps are involved in the extraction of leads from a superior access site via the implant vein:

1. Pocket access: Once the CIED pocket has been opened, leads are carefully freed from anchoring sites including the removal of suture sleeves, suture material and any fibrotic binding sites as close to the actual venous entry site as feasible to allow for effective and coaxial maneuverability of the extraction sheaths. Preplacement of a purse-string suture with a Rummel tourniquet at this point is advisable to prevent significant intraprocedural and postprocedural blood loss (**Fig. 2**). If infection is suspected, capsule debridement should be completed and culture swabs and debrided pocket material sent for microbiological analysis.
2. Lead preparation for explant: Leads are disconnected from the generator and then loaded with a stylet for support. In case of selective lead removal, stylets should still be introduced into the remaining leads to reduce the risk of lead dislodgment. Any active fixation lead mechanism should be retracted with the manufacturer's wrench or a curved hemostat for better grip. Additional lead body rotations can be

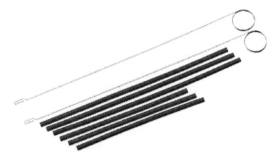

Fig. 2. Rummel tourniquet, used to prevent backbleeding from implant venous site. (*Courtesy of* Medtronic, Inc., Minneapolis, MN; with permission. © Medtronic 2018.)

attempted if the fixation helix does not initially retract. Retraction of the helical screw may be more effective if the lead is cut and the inner coil exposed and the standard stylet inserted to the tip if possible.

3. Simple manual traction can then be attempted to remove the lead under fluoroscopic guidance. Although this is usually the situation for leads implanted less than 1 year, even leads implanted for short periods can become densely adherent to the veins of cardiac chambers and require lead extraction set-up and tools.
4. Lead preparation for extraction: If simple explant attempts fail, specialized tools should be used for extraction starting with placement of a lead locking device. A variety of lead locking devices are available. The Cook Liberator locking stylet locks only at the distal tip and does not allow repositioning once locked. The Spectranetics (Colorado Springs, CO) lead locking devices allow for locking along the entire lead body and come in different lengths and varying tensile strengths. The lead header connectors are generally cut medial to any connector bifurcation. When dealing with a defibrillator lead, the outer insulation of the lead is carefully removed with a scalpel exposing the conductor coil and shock coil cables. A locking stylet is then introduced and locked as far distal toward the lead tip as possible to avoid creating a proximal predetermined breaking point between locked and unlocked lead portions. When it is difficult to advance the locking stylet, a clearing stylet can sometimes be helpful to clear the path. Once locked in place, the lead's remaining components including outer insulation and shock coil cable are then secured to the proximal end of the locking stylet with additional suture ties of high tensile strength to avoid separation and unraveling during extraction.

We use Supramid suture (S. Jackson Inc, Alexandria, VA), a nylon monofilament suture that has higher tensile strength than other nonabsorbable synthetic suture materials and creates slimmer knots than braided materials such as Ethibond (Johnson & Johnson Medical NV, Diegem, Belgium). This ensures that the different lead components do not separate and remain in the vasculature during the extraction process (**Fig. 3**). Once adequately locked and secured, careful manual traction is again used to extract the lead.

5. Use of specialized extraction sheaths: If mild manual traction remains unsuccessful, the use of specialized extraction sheaths is required. For initial access to the venous insertion site in a tight fibrotic or calcified area around the costoclavicular space, a mechanical rotational dissection sheath is most helpful (Evolution RL/RL Shortie, Cook Medical, Bloomington, IN; TightRail Sub-C, Spectranetics) (**Fig. 4**). Alternatively, telescoping sheaths of different materials can be used to overcome heavy fibrous calcifications. Once the venous access site has been freed of adhesions and is accessible, the mechanical sheath is frequently exchanged for a laser sheath after appropriate sizing and calibration (CVX-300 Excimer Laser and Glidelight/SLS II Laser Sheath, Spectranetics) (**Fig. 5**). Application of sterile light mineral oil can be helpful to decrease friction between the lead-stylet-suture assembly and the inner surface of the laser sheath allowing for better maneuverability of the laser sheath and more refined control over manually applied counterpressure. When advancing the laser sheath, it is critical that (1) well-balanced (firm but not too firm) traction be applied to the lead-stylet assembly combined with slow rotational motion of the laser or mechanical sheath to allow for mechanical dilation while maintaining as coaxial a rail as possible; (2) laser energy should be applied only when the sheath cannot easily be advanced by hand; and (3) the laser sheath's beveled edge be kept on the lesser curvature of the brachiocephalic venous course

to avoid avulsion or perforation into the free mediastinal space (**Fig. 6**).

6. Overcoming significant fibrous adhesions: When the laser sheath does not advance despite application of laser energy and appropriate counterpressure, this may indicate more robust binding sites containing calcification. These are typically present in the costoclavicular area, SVC, at the junction of right atrium and inferior vena cava (IVC), and at the tricuspid valve level. In these scenarios, multiple exchanges between laser and mechanical rotational tools may lead to success. "Snow plowing" of material in front of the sheath tip may require an upgrade to a larger sheath size. As the sheath nears the tip of the lead, a final apical binding site can usually be freed successfully with gentle countertraction, sometimes steadily held over several minutes and avoiding overzealous traction (see **Fig. 6**; **Figs. 7** and **8**).

7. Lead retrieval: Once the lead has been freed of any binding sites, it can be removed by simple traction through the laser or mechanical sheath. With attention to avoid blood loss or air embolism, the sheath then serves as a vascular access conduit, through which a guide wire can be immediately advanced to maintain vascular access, and the sheath is removed. The explanted lead should always be inspected for clues of perforation, such as presence of adipose tissue on the lead tip (see **Fig. 8**).

8. Pocket management: Following lead retrieval, attention should then be directed to hemostasis at the venous access site using the initially prepared purse-string suture and in the device pocket itself followed by implant of a new device, if indicated, and pocket closure. In case of manifest or suspected infections, after careful pocket revision and debridement, we often use wound vacuum-assisted therapy to promote tissue granulation in conjunction with local and systemic antibiotics and delayed primary closure strategy. If the area of skin excised is relatively small, many centers debride the pocket of all nonviable or infected tissue, obtain hemostasis, and provide primary

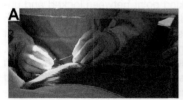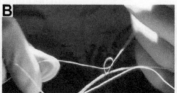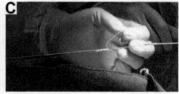

Fig. 3. After the lead has been cut, a locking stylet is introduced into the lead lumen (*A*). The outer insulation is then secured to the lead body (*B*) and the locking stylet (*C*) with Supramid suture. Additional suture ties are needed for further lead components in the case of a defibrillator lead.

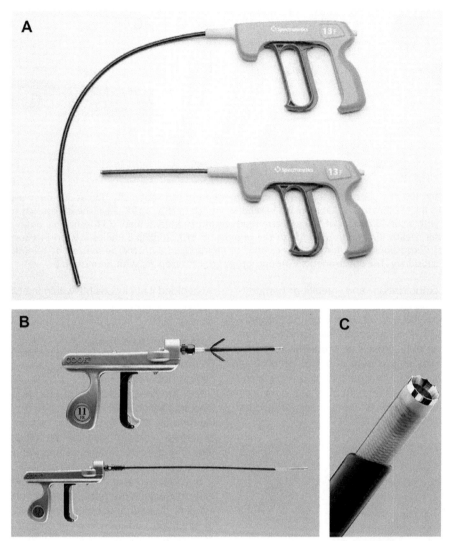

Fig. 4. Mechanical rotational extraction tools. (*A*) TightRail (*top*) and TightRail Sub-C (*bottom*); (*B*) Evolution RL (*bottom*) and Shortie RL (*top*) Shortie. (*C*) Rotational motion of a low-profile blade dissects tissue at the tip of the sheath. ([*A*] *Reproduced with the permission* of Koninklijke Philips N.V. and its subsidiary, The Spectranetics Corporation. All rights reserved; [*B*] Permission for use granted by Cook Medical, Bloomington, Indiana; and [*C*] *Courtesy of* Cook Medical, Bloomington, IN; with permission.)

closure with interrupted vertical mattress sutures, with or without a closed drainage system.

Special Considerations and Limitations in Superior Extractions Via the Implant Vein

1. When multiple leads are extracted, the most recently implanted lead should be removed first, as it will likely be easier to extract. When stalled progression occurs at fibrotic lead-lead binding sites, turning attention to the other lead in an alternating approach is more likely going to result in success (see **Fig. 6**). Upsizing the sheath from 14-French to 16-French in conjunction with an outer sheath may be necessary to provide additional mechanical advantage and overcome a "snow-plowing" effect of lead insulation or fibrous tissue (see **Fig. 5B**).

2. In the removal of infected systems in which vegetations are adherent to leads, upsizing to a larger 16-French sheath may be necessary to extract the lead in its entirety while avoiding shearing off vegetation material. The Angiovac system (AngioDynamics, Latham, NY) can reduce embolization when the burden of vegetations is large (**Fig. 9**).[9,10] When vegetations are exceptionally sizable (>2–3 cm), transvenous removal is discouraged due to the risk of

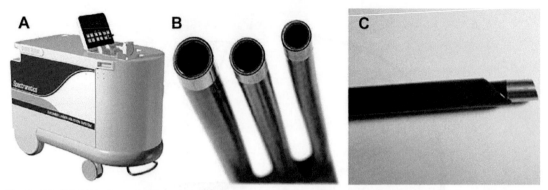

Fig. 5. (*A*) CVX-300, the generator that emits an excimer laser using xenon-chloride at 308-nm wavelength. (*B*) Glidelight/SLS II laser sheaths available in 16, 14, and 12 French (*left to right*). Each sheath consists of 82 optical fibers, each with a core diameter of 100 μm, arranged around an inner lumen. (*C*) Mechanical outer sheath over the inner laser sheath. ([*A*] *Reproduced with the permission* of Koninklijke Philips N.V. and its subsidiary, The Spectranetics Corporation. All rights reserved; and [*B*] *Reproduced with the permission of* Koninklijke Philips N.V. and its subsidiary, The Spectranetics Corporation. All rights reserved; with permission.)

saddle embolization and resulting hemodynamic collapse.

3. Left ventricular lead removal from the coronary sinus (CS) is approached similarly to other leads and may present a problem, as adhesions to other leads or the CS body itself commonly exist. Removal techniques are identical to those used for right atrial and right ventricular leads, however, laser energy should be avoided if at all possible within the CS given the risk of dissection.

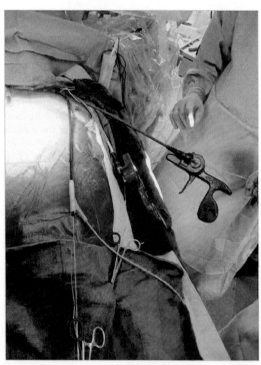

Fig. 6. Laser and mechanical sheaths being advanced over multiple lead-stylet-suture assemblies simultaneously.

Commonly Used Tools

Locking stylets (Lead Locking Device, Spectranetics; Liberator Beacon Tip Locking Stylet, Cook Medical). Locking stylets add essential lead stability and tensile strength to the lead allowing for manual traction, countertraction, and maintaining a coaxial rail for extraction sheaths, reducing the risk of lead disintegration (**Fig. 10, Table 1**).

Bulldog lead extender (Cook Medical). A lead extender aids in the removal of lumenless cardiac leads or those that contain cable conductor wires by anchoring on the proximal portion of the lead and allowing extraction sheaths to be threaded over the lead extender–lead assembly (**Fig. 11**).

Rummel tourniquet (Medtronic, Minneapolis, MN, USA and other various suppliers). A Rummel tourniquet is helpful in achieving intraprocedural and postprocedural hemostasis, especially when multiple sheath exchanges with varying diameters are required. It is threaded over a purse-string suture initially placed around the implant venous access site. The compression of the purse-string suture can then be adjusted with a hemostat (see **Fig. 1**).

Supramid suture (S. Jackson Inc). Supramid suture is a nylon monofilament suture with higher tensile strength than other nonabsorbable synthetic suture materials and creates slimmer knots than braided materials. It is used to connect the outer lead insulation and shock coil wires with the locking stylet and prevents unraveling from the lead's core during extraction (see **Fig. 3**).

One-Tie Compression Coil (Cook Medical). A One-Tie Compression Coil is intended to be used

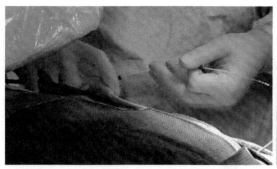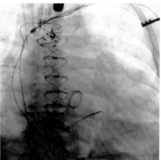

Fig. 7. Laser sheath being advanced under fluoroscopic guidance.

to aid in the removal of an implantable cardiac lead by binding the proximal components of the lead together and to an engaged locking stylet or to an affixed lead extender (**Fig. 12**). This is particularly useful, and is used in addition to the locking stylets, in leads that are fragile and more elastic in properties.

Mechanical rotational extraction tools. The TightRail and TightRail Sub-C (Spectranetics) (see **Fig. 4**A); Evolution RL/Shortie RL (Cook Medical) (see **Fig. 4**B). Mechanical rotational extraction tools allow for dissection of tissue at the tip of the sheath through the rotational motion of a low-profile blade (see **Fig. 4**C). These devices can be especially helpful to advance through heavily fibrosed or calcified areas.

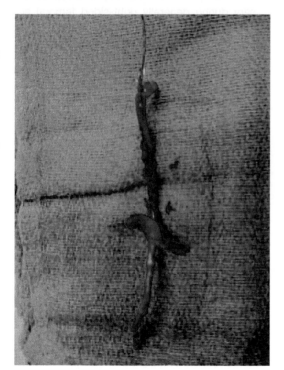

Fig. 8. Fibrotic adhesions and myocardial tissue attached to extracted right ventricular lead.

Laser extraction tool (CVX-300 Excimer Laser and Glidelight/SLS II Laser Sheaths, Spectranetics). The laser sheath advances through tissue using 135 ns pulsed xenon-chloride laser-emitting light with a wavelength of 308 nm at a repetition rate of 25 to 80 Hz. Absorption of the laser energy is 95% at 0.18-mm depth. The energy is absorbed by lipids and proteins but not by water, enabling the laser to preferentially disrupt fibrotic tissue (see **Fig. 5**).

Telescoping Sheaths

Telescoping sheaths are available in different materials, including Teflon, polypropylene, or stainless steel, with the corresponding variations in stiffness and ability to dissect adhesions. Available products include the SightRail Manual Dilator Sheath Set (Spectranetics) and the Byrd Dilator Sheaths Telescoping PTFE, Byrd Dilator Sheaths Telescoping Polypropylene, and Byrd Dilator Sheaths Telescoping Stainless Steel (Cook Medical).

Occlusion Balloon (Bridge Occlusion Balloon, Spectranetics). A tear in the SVC during a lead extraction procedure is a rare, but life-threatening event. A guidewire is placed from the right femoral vein extending to the right internal jugular vein before advancing laser or mechanical sheaths. A highly compliant 8-cm occlusion balloon can be quickly deployed over the guidewire and placed across the SVC to reduce blood loss through an SVC tear, reduce the rate of hemorrhage, and allow time for transition to surgical repair (**Fig. 13**).

Angiovac (AngioDynamics). In the presence of significant infective vegetations, use of the Angiovac system can be considered to reduce the risk of embolization to the pulmonary artery bed (see **Fig. 9**).

FEMORAL APPROACH

Femoral vein access is a versatile yet complex approach for lead removal and essential in various scenarios[5,6]:

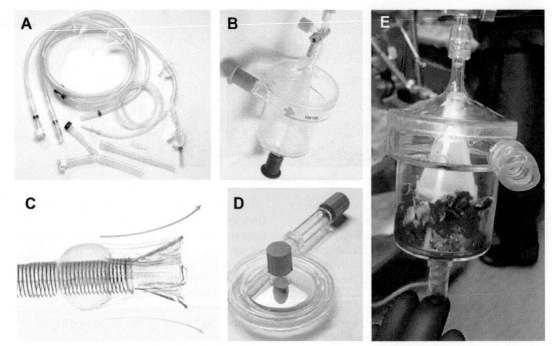

Fig. 9. Angiovac system to reduce the risk of embolization to the pulmonary bed. (*A*) Angiovac circuit tubing. (*B*) Filter and bubble trap to collect thrombus/vegetation material. (*C*) Cannula and obturator. (*D*) Maquet pump head. (*E*) Extracted material. (*Courtesy of* AngioDynamics, Latham, NY; with permission.)

- Extraction of purposefully cut leads or lead fragments, including previously abandoned leads that have retracted into the proximal vasculature.
- Leads that have conductors without a lumen or otherwise do not accept a locking stylet are more difficult to remove from a progressive dissection superior approach due to decreased tensile strength and relative coaxial instability resulting in disintegration or accordioning/snow plowing of the insulation of the lead.
- Leads requiring distal support to maintain coaxial stability for combined superior access tools, including when venous access needs to be maintained due to venous obstruction.
- Leads implanted via the femoral route are more easily removed via the original route of implant.
- Nonavailability of superior access extraction systems.
- Failure of superior access lead extraction.

Technique

The femoral extraction approach consists of several steps:

1. Femoral vein access: The Byrd Femoral Work Station (Cook Medical) is an invaluable and

the most commonly used tool used in femoral extractions (**Fig. 14**). Careful attention is necessary during generally right-sided femoral access and while upsizing to a 16-French caliber sheath to avoid vascular complications. The sheath is then advanced to the lower right atrium or IVC such that additional tools can be inserted and used through the workstation. A side port present on the 16-French sheath can be used for irrigation and thrombus prevention. Use of pressurized heparinized saline to keep the large lumen flushed is useful.

2. Lead preparation: When femoral extraction becomes necessary, proximal lead portions are often unavailable for insertion of locking stylets or retraction of an active fixation helix at the distal lead tip. Cut leads should be freed up proximally from any anchoring forces, including suture sleeves and surrounding fibrous tissue to facilitate removal via femoral traction. When a combined superior and femoral approach is planned, locking stylets may already be in place and provide additional tensile strength for subsequent femoral removal. Certain situations may favor a more floppy lead when the use of locking stylets with unlocking and repositioning ability (Lead Locking Device, Spectranetics) can be considered (see **Fig. 10**).[5] However, the lack of tensile reinforcement during

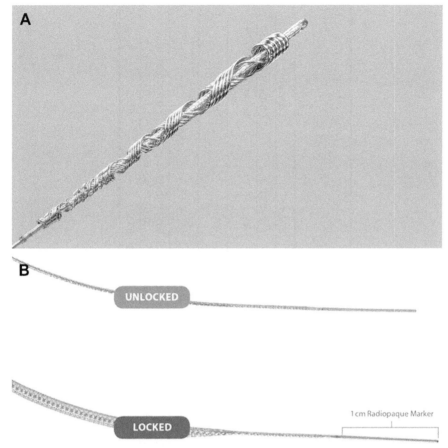

Fig. 10. Locking stylets and mechanisms. ([*A*] *Permission for* use granted by Cook Medical, Bloomington, Indiana; and [*B*] *Reproduced with the permission of* Koninklijke Philips N.V. and its subsidiary, The Spectranetics Corporation. All rights reserved.)

application of traction forces on the lead can result in its disintegration ("unraveling") more often so during femoral than superior approach.

3. Mechanical lead capture: The 16-French sheath is a conduit for additional extraction tools and serves as a counterpressure and countertraction device. Depending on the clinical scenario, a telescoping sheath and a combination of deflecting wires, guide and deflectable catheters, helical loop (Dotter) basket, bioptome, gooseneck, and needle's-eye snares are used to stabilize and mechanically capture the lead. Generally, when either the proximal free end or distal electrode tip of the lead is available, a gooseneck snare or bioptome are used to grasp it. When no free end is available, a needle's-eye snare, deflectable guidewire, or a catheter can be used (see **Fig. 14**; **Figs. 15–17**). If a deflecting guidewire is used, a basket, snare, or other device that can be closed over the guidewire will entrap the lead for subsequent removal.

4. Overcoming significant fibrous adhesions: When fibrous adhesions are significant and not overcome by traction maneuvers within the subclavian vein or SVC, the use of radiofrequency (RF) ablation catheters has been suggested and successfully used by some centers to make the lead available for grasping or free it for further traction attempts.[5] In such cases, even right internal jugular access can prove useful to reach challenging locations or to remove a lead via an alternate route. Furthermore, femoral extractions using laser sheaths have been successfully used in some cases, limited in reach by a sheath length originally designed and approved for superior access at the implant vein site.

5. Lead retrieval: On successful capture of the lead, the femoral workstation's inner 12-French telescoping sheath is advanced toward the distal end of the grasping tool to further stabilize the lead and secure the capture point at the lead. The telescoping sheath is then

Table 1
Overview of available locking stylets and individual features

Feature	Spectranetics					Cook
	LLD EZ	LLD E	LLD #1	LLD #2	LLD #3	Liberator
Model number	518–062	518–039	518–018	518–019	518–020	LR-OFA0I/G26550
Locks along entire lead lumen	Yes	Yes	Yes	Yes	Yes	Locks the distal 3 inches
May unlock and be repositioned	Yes	Yes	Yes	Yes	Yes	No
Average tensile strength,[a] lb	19	19	12	24	45	14
Locking range, diameter, mm	0.015*/0.38 to 0.023*/0.58	0.015*/0.38 to 0.023*/0.58	0.013*/0.33 to 0.016*/0.41	0.017*/0.43 to 0.026*/0.66	0.027*/0.69 to 0.032*/0.81	0.016*/0.41 to 0.032*/0.81
Working length, cm	65	85	65	65	65	70

[a] Minimum specification for LLD EZ, LLD E, LLD #2, and LLD #3 is 10 lb; minimum for LLD #1 is 7 lb.

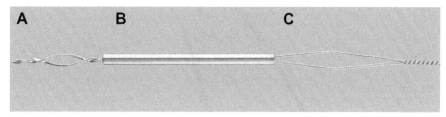

Fig. 11. Bulldog lead extender. The smaller aperture provides anchoring site to tie outer portion of lead to the lead extender (A); advancing metal sleeve closes larger aperture and secures exposed lead in place during removal (B); larger aperture allows capture of exposed lead or cable conductors (C). (*Courtesy of* Cook Medical, Bloomington, IN; with permission.)

withdrawn into the outer 16-French sheath by careful traction maneuvers. When the distal tip of the lead is still attached to apical myocardium, the free end of the lead can be externalized followed by advancement of a mechanical telescoping sheath toward the distal end to carefully break up additional adhesions at the myocardial lead interface by traction and the countertraction technique. Managing the workstation's stiff extraction sheaths can prove especially challenging at the sharp turn across the tricuspid valve. Once the lead has been freed, it can usually be pulled into the IVC within the 16-French outer sheath for final retrieval.

6. Sheath removal and hemostasis: We routinely place a figure-8 stitch on removal of the 16-French femoral venous sheath. The stitch approximates a bundle of soft tissue overlying and compressing the venotomy site, resulting in highly effective hemostasis and reducing bleeding complications.[11]

Special Considerations and Limitations in Femoral Lead Extractions

1. Mobilized leads occasionally have abundant fibrous material adhered making externalization through the 16-French femoral workstation impossible. In such cases, femoral venous cut-down and vascular repair may be required.[5]

2. The great versatility of tools used in femoral extractions may make dislodgment of nontargeted leads more likely, and consideration for placement of a transvenous pacing wire should be considered in pacemaker-dependent patients.

3. CS leads are amenable to extraction via the femoral approach when no adhesions have formed within the CS; for example, using a needle's-eye snare.

4. Given the manipulation of tools in a 3-dimensional space, particularly during the femoral approach, procedure time is longer, resulting in increased radiation exposure for both patient and operator, and careful consideration should be placed on adequate shielding and fluoroscopy practice.[6]

5. Femoral extraction is contraindicated when an IVC filter is in place due to the potential for perforation of the vascular wall when traction is applied on the limbs of the filter.

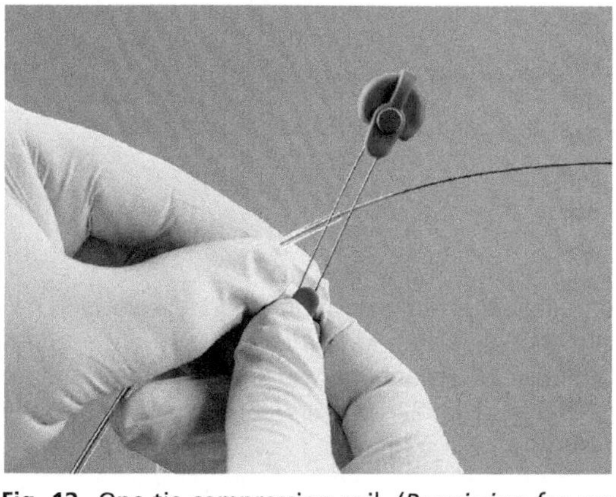

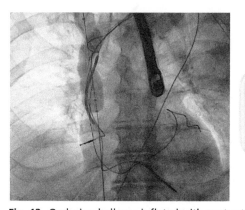

Fig. 12. One-tie compression coil. (*Permission for* use granted by Cook Medical, Bloomington, Indiana.)

Fig. 13. Occlusion balloon, inflated with contrast dye to visualize position in the SVC. (*Permission for* use granted by Cook Medical, Bloomington, Indiana.)

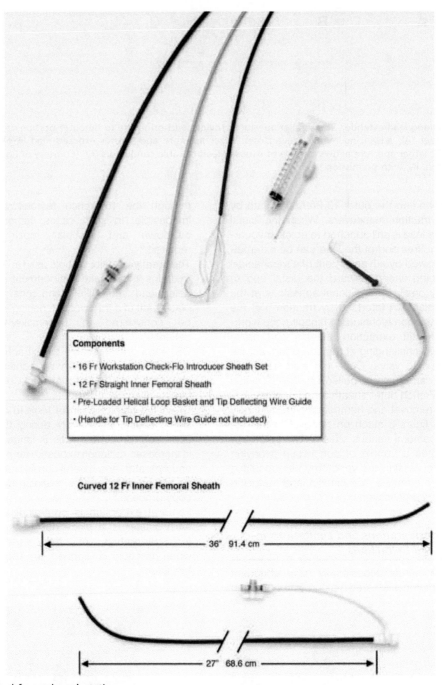

Components

• 16 Fr Workstation Check-Flo Introducer Sheath Set

• 12 Fr Straight Inner Femoral Sheath

• Pre-Loaded Helical Loop Basket and Tip Deflecting Wire Guide

• (Handle for Tip Deflecting Wire Guide not included)

Curved 12 Fr Inner Femoral Sheath

← 36" 91.4 cm →

← 27" 68.6 cm →

Fig. 14. Byrd femoral work station.

Commonly Used Tools

The Byrd femoral workstation (Cook Medical) is the most commonly used tool for extraction using the femoral approach. Essential parts of the set include a 16-French workstation introducer sheath with a side port for continuous irrigation and prevention of thrombus formation, a 12-French straight inner femoral sheath, and a preloaded helical loop basket and tip deflecting wire guide. An optional 12-French curved inner femoral sheath is included in 27-inch and 36-inch lengths (see **Fig. 14**).

The needle's-eye snare (Cook Medical) comes in combination with the previously described

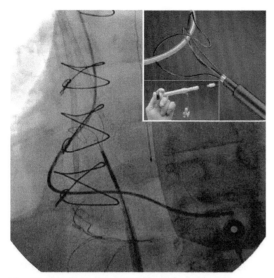

Fig. 15. Needle's-eye snare grasping lead body when no free end of lead is available. (*Courtesy of* Cook Medical, Bloomington, IN; with permission.)

workstation components or as a single device and is available in a 13-mm and 20-mm profile size. The larger size is useful for capture of larger caliber (defibrillator) leads (see **Fig. 15**).

Gooseneck snares (various suppliers) form a loop coming perpendicular off the shaft and thus stay coaxial to the vessel lumen. Various loop diameters are available. Most commonly used sizes range from 5 to 25 mm and additional smaller microsnares (see **Fig. 16**A; various suppliers).

Gastric or cardiac bioptomes (various suppliers) are helpful to grasp lead-retained lead fragments and in clinical scenarios similar to when other grasping tools, such as snares and helical loop basket catheters, are used (see **Fig. 17**).

Guide catheters and deflectable wire guides (various suppliers) are helpful when orienting 3-dimensional tools in relation a lead target under fluoroscopy, as they can add additional directional information and be used to drag leads toward the snare (see **Fig. 16**B).

Deflectable ablation catheters (various suppliers) can be used to form a robust and adjustable hook mechanism to drag a lead to the snare. Some centers use RF ablation energy to free leads from adhesions.[6]

SURGICAL MANAGEMENT

Despite diligent preparation and procedure execution in an experienced center, life-threatening complications, including peripheral and central vascular complications, as well as myocardial tears, may occur. Although an SVC occlusion balloon can temporize central venous complications, swift transition to open surgical management is imperative.

Surgical management of lead extractions is also indicated in the presence of a large burden of infective vegetation material. Our institution favors surgical lead extractions when vegetation dimensions exceed 3 cm, posing a risk for hemodynamically relevant pulmonary embolization. Furthermore, transition to surgical management may become necessary when transvenous lead extraction fails and retained leads or lead fragments require removal based on the underlying clinical circumstances. The reader is referred to the articles on surgical management elsewhere in this issue.

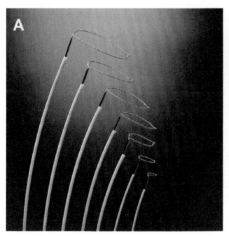
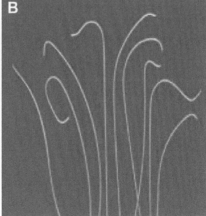

Fig. 16. Femoral tools including gooseneck snares (*A*) and guide catheters (*B*). (*Permission for* use granted by Cook Medical, Bloomington, Indiana.)

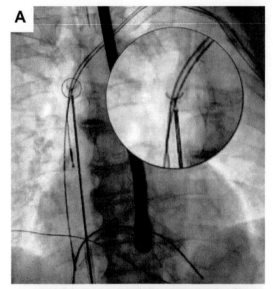

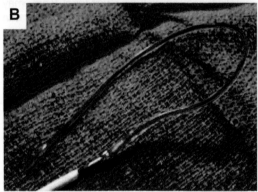

Fig. 17. (*A*) Gastric bioptome grasping lead body. (*B*) Postextraction bioptome and lead. (*From* Fischer A, Pretorius V, Birgersdotter-Green U. Femoral lead extraction: an underappreciated and underutilized approach to lead removal. The Journal of Innovations in Cardiac Rhythm Management. 2012;3:682–7; with permission.)

SUMMARY

The complex skillset required for transvenous lead removal is in growing demand along with increasing numbers of implanted CIEDs. A systematic and comprehensive approach, including knowledge of all available tools and vascular access techniques is essential for successful outcomes.

REFERENCES

1. Varajan SL, Pretorius V, Birgersdotter-Green U. Transvenous lead extraction: a step-by-step approach. J Innovations Card Rhythm Manage 2011;145–9.

2. Kusumoto FM, Schoenfeld MH, Wilkoff BL, et al. HRS expert consensus statement on cardiovascular implantable electronic device lead management and extraction. Heart Rhythm 2017;14(12): e503–51.

3. Wilkoff BL, Love CJ, Byrd CL, et al. Transvenous lead extraction: heart rhythm society expert consensus on facilities, training, indications, and patient management: this document was endorsed by the American Heart Association (AHA). Heart Rhythm 2009;6(7):1085–104.

4. Diemberger I, Mazzotti A, Giulia MB, et al. From lead management to implanted patient management: systematic review and meta-analysis of the last 15 years of experience in lead extraction. Expert Rev Med Devices 2013;10(4):551–73.

5. Mulpuru SK, Hayes DL, Osborn MJ, et al. Femoral approach to lead extraction. J Cardiovasc Electrophysiol 2015;26(3):357–61.

6. Fischer A, Pretorius V, Birdersdotter-Green U. Femoral lead extraction: an underappreciated and underutilized approach to lead removal. J Innovations Card Rhythm Manage 2012;682–7.

7. Bordachar P, Defaye P, Peyrouse E, et al. Extraction of old pacemaker or cardioverter-defibrillator leads by laser sheath versus femoral approach. Circ Arrhythm Electrophysiol 2010;3(4):319–23.

8. Bongiorni MG, Kennergren C, Butter C, et al. The European lead extraction controlled (ELECTRa) study: a European Heart Rhythm Association (EHRA) registry of transvenous lead extraction outcomes. Eur Heart J 2017;38(40): 2995–3005.

9. Edla S, Boshara A, Neupane S, et al. Internal jugular venous approach to percutaneous vacuum-assisted debulking of large lead vegetations prior to lead extraction. JACC Clin Electrophysiol 2018;4(1):147–8.

10. Patel N, Azemi T, Zaeem F, et al. Vacuum assisted vegetation extraction for the management of large lead vegetations. J Card Surg 2013;28(3):321–4.

11. Lakshmanadoss U, Wong WS, Kutinsky I, et al. Figure-of-eight suture for venous hemostasis in fully anticoagulated patients after atrial fibrillation catheter ablation. Indian Pacing Electrophysiol J 2017; 17(5):134–9.

Cardiac and Vascular Injuries Sustained During Transvenous Lead Extraction

Jamil Bashir, MD, FRCS(C)[a],*,
Roger G. Carrillo, MD, MBA, FHRS[b]

KEYWORDS

- Cardiac surgery • Cardiac tamponade • Cardiopulmonary bypass • Laser • Lead extraction
- Pacemaker

KEY POINTS

- Venous or cardiac injury in the setting of transvenous lead extraction is a devastating complication with a high mortality.
- The immediate availability of cardiac surgical back-up with the ability to implement cardiopulmonary bypass is by far the safest environment for lead extraction.
- Repair techniques are reproducible and should be widely disseminated and understood in institutions where extraction is performed.

INTRODUCTION

The rapid rise in indications for cardiac implantable electronic devices has necessitated the development of tools for removal of the electrodes that connect the heart to these externally located pacemakers and defibrillators. Almost immediately after the implant of a cardiac electrode, there is clear evidence of the development of fibrous attachments to the heart and vascular structures that they traverse.[1] The natural history of this fibrosis is one of variable but progressive fibrous adhesion. Eventually, most electrodes develop strong fibrous attachments at the point of entry to the vein, areas of contact within veins they traverse, the tricuspid valve, and finally in the area of contact within cardiac chambers that are sensed and paced.[2]

These adhesions have a few fundamental properties that directly impact extraction and potential complications:

1. The adhesion can be stronger than the tissue it adheres to such that simply pulling on the electrode damages the electrode or tears/damages normal tissue before the electrode comes free[2]
2. Calcification of the adhesions frequently occurs as they age
3. Adhesions in general become denser as they age but are highly variable from person to person[3]

The nature of these adhesions has precipitated the development of powerful tools that can cut fibrous tissue and calcified fibrous tissue to free electrodes for a variety of critical reasons, such

Disclosure Statement: J. Bashir: The author has active research grants from Boston Scientific and Spectranetics. These are arm's length grants. The author is a consultant for Boston Scientific. R.G. Carrillo: The author has research grants from Abbott, Medtronic, Boston Scientific, Tyco, and Spectranetics.
a University of British Columbia, St. Paul's Hospital, Room 458, 4th Floor, Burrard Building, 1081 Burrard Street, Vancouver, British Columbia V6Z 1Y6, Canada; b University of Miami, Miller School of Medicine, 1295 Northwest 14 Street, Suite H, Miami, FL 33125, USA
* Corresponding author.
E-mail address: jmlbashir@gmail.com

Card Electrophysiol Clin 10 (2018) 651–657
https://doi.org/10.1016/j.ccep.2018.08.003

as infection. These tools, and the mechanical tools that preceded them, can also cut through normal vascular and cardiac tissue and therefore carry a well-described risk of full-thickness disruption of the veins or heart. These injuries generally lead to cardiac tamponade or right hemothorax depending on the location of injury. They are potentially devastating complications with a high risk of mortality if not treated surgically in a highly expeditious and appropriate manner.[4] This article describes the incidence, risk factors, and diagnosis of these injuries followed by discussion of recent evidence for the use of superior vena cava (SVC) balloon occlusion and finally, conventional surgical repair of these injuries.

INCIDENCE OF CARDIAC AND VASCULAR INJURY

The published incidence of these injuries varies widely. A multicenter study of mostly highly experienced extractors in the Lexicon study revealed a combined cardiac or vascular avulsion rate of 1.0% and many other expert single centers and operators have also published rates of injury that are low and around 1%.[5–7] However, population-level data from British Columbia revealed a 3% rate of injury from three centers performing extraction and other series including the early European experience have reported even higher rates.[8–11] Unfortunately, extraction injuries are not tracked in a systematic fashion and there is no clear understanding of the population level rate of injury in large regions, such as the United States or Europe. Concerns regarding a higher than expected rate of injury and death because of these injuries came from an original provocative study from Hauser and colleagues[4] that revealed 105 injuries reported to the MAUDE database from 1995 to 2008. A recent review of injuries from only one manufacturer of lead extraction tools within the MAUDE database revealed 68 injuries within a 6-month period in 2016. This leads us to believe that at least 200 potentially fatal injuries occur per year in the United States, and (with an assumed rate of 10,000 extractions per year) a 2% rate of perforation is possible.[12]

Ultimately, the absolute rate of injury is secondary to the level of preparedness of the center performing the extraction because patients undergoing extraction will continue to be exposed to this risk for the foreseeable future.

RISK FACTORS FOR PERFORATION

The ability to predict in a general sense that a given patient is at an increased risk for an operative event could be highly beneficial in enhancing operative planning and is a commonly used strategy in cardiac surgery (Euroscore II, STS score).[13,14] Many studies have attempted to determine the risk factors associated with major complications including avulsion or perforation injuries at the time of extraction. The relative scarcity of injuries has made evaluation of associated variables difficult as has the paucity of large studies that evaluate enough patients with these complications. Authors have in some ways compounded this problem by grouping outcomes into categories that may not in fact be related even though this was likely done to gain statistical significance. An example is the confounding between mortality and perforation: although perforation may be a significant risk for mortality, they are distinct outcomes. Mortality is associated with extraction for other reasons, such as infection. In the Lexicon study, the outcome of extraction in 1449 patients was analyzed as "major adverse events" to group enough events together for analysis.[7]

There is significant controversy regarding which variables impart a higher risk of perforation and not all of them are described as concretely imparting increased risk. The main variables that have previously been hypothesized to be associated with cardiac or vascular perforation are included in **Box 1**.[15]

Since the earliest analyses of lead extraction complications, female gender has been deemed a significant risk factor for major complications including perforation. In the original review of extractions performed between 1994 and 1996, women had a statistically significant higher rate

---

Box 1
Variables associated with perforation

a. Female gender

b. Operator experience

c. Superior vena cava high-voltage coil

d. Age of leads or dwell time in body

e. Powered sheaths

f. Femoral approach

g. Lack of previous open-heart surgery

h. Internal cardioverter defibrillator leads

i. Increased number of leads extracted

From Kusumoto FM, Schoenfeld MH, Wilkoff BL, et al. 2017 HRS expert consensus statement on cardiovascular implantable electronic device lead management and extraction. Heart Rhythm 2017;14(12):e503–51; with permission.

of "major complications" at 1.9% (0.7% for men).[16] This increased to 8.6% and was highly significant if women with more than three leads were compared with men (1.5%). Subsequent analyses including our own population-based analysis of all extraction injuries in British Columbia revealed a highly significant increased risk for women as did the Electra registry.[8,17,18]

Operator experience is a frequently discussed factor that is clearly associated with procedural success and risk of complications.[16–18] This is an intuitive finding but also complex in its effect because poor technique could easily lead to inadvertent injury and the interplay with other risk factors is not clear. The most recent study focusing on experience was the large prospective European Electra registry, which found a lower rate of all-cause complications in high-volume centers. There was a strong trend toward an increase in procedure-related complications in low-volume centers but this did not reach statistical significance. Techniques used for extraction in this study were highly heterogeneous because traction alone was used in 27.3% and powered sheaths in only 27.1%, which makes it generalizable to larger populations but not specific.

A convincing research letter published from a group of experienced extractors revealed concrete evidence of a higher rate of perforation with the presence of an SVC coil and this finding has been reproduced in other single-center series.[19,20]

Lead age seems to be one of the most powerful predictors of difficult and complicated extractions because it has a proven direct impact on the density of electrode adhesion and the presence of calcification.[3] Many studies have found this to be an important predictor of the need for advanced extraction tools and techniques and increased risk of complications.[17,18] In the ELECTRA registry, leads with a dwell time of more than 10 years had a highly significant increased risk of major complications with an odds ratio of 3.54.

The use of a powered sheath has been reproducibly associated with major complications and perforations in particular.[18,20] These tools are readily able to cut through normal vessel walls or tissue and in area where the lead is tightly adherent to a thin vessel wall, the tool can cut the vessel open and allow blood to enter the pericardium or pleural space.

The femoral approach has also been associated with injury risk in large studies, although this has not been a universal finding.[18] A small randomized trial and observational study found no difference between the techniques but was likely underpowered.[21] The number of leads extracted has been associated with extraction risk in at least two studies[10,16] but this has frequently been confounded by other risk factors, such as female gender (see previously).

Ultimately, registry data that involve much larger sample sizes are required to create an operative risk score similar to ones available for cardiovascular surgery. There is tremendous complexity in the interplay between experience (technique) and multiple factors that may individually impart risk. Risk scoring, indeed, is entirely historical and can only describe the event rate of previous patient groups under similar circumstances.

DIAGNOSIS OF INJURY

The mechanism of disruption of normal physiology by vascular and cardiac injuries depends on a host of factors including the location, size of injury, chamber affected, and central venous pressure.[8,9,22] However, there are only a few final common pathways by which the problem manifests and either cardiac tamponade (84.8% in our series[8]) or right hemothorax predominate, although other mechanisms are rarely possible. In SVC injuries, the location could be extrapericardial, presenting usually as a right hemothorax, or intrapericardial, presenting as cardiac tamponade. The pericardial reflection covers up to 40% of the SVC (**Fig. 1**). In all cases, hypotension as a result of low cardiac output is a salient feature and in severe injury this is sudden, severe, and, if protracted, irreversible without surgical rescue. The gold standard for diagnosis of cardiac tamponade is transesophageal echocardiography. Anecdotally, we have found that an immobile cardiac shadow on fluoroscopy (especially if leads are still present and moving internally) is also a highly sensitive test for tamponade (**Fig. 2**). Right hemothorax

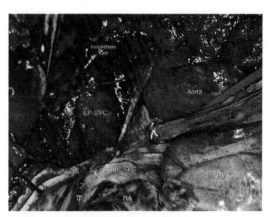

Fig. 1. Intraoperative photograph showing anatomy of the superior vena cava. EP-SVC, extrapericardial superior vena cava; IP-SVC, intrapericardial superior vena cava; RA, right atrium; RV, right ventricle.

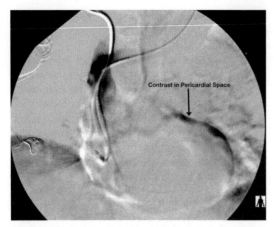

Fig. 2. Fluoroscopy showing intrapericardial superior vena cava tear with contrast extravagating into pericardial space.

may also be diagnosed with transesophageal echocardiography, which reveals an empty normal contracting ventricle and a large right pleural effusion. Right hemothorax can also be evident on fluoroscopy where the right hemothorax has more density than the left.

OCCLUSION BALLOON
Description and Usage

The occlusion balloon is a rescue tool used in the event of SVC tears to provide hemostasis at the site of injury. It is a compliant, low-pressure plastic balloon that is 80 mm in length and 20 mm in diameter and has a maximum inflation volume of 60 mL. In the event of a sudden patient hypotension during a lead extraction procedure, the balloon can be rapidly deployed to the site of injury and inflated to prevent excessive blood loss before a surgical repair is initiated (**Fig. 3**).[12]

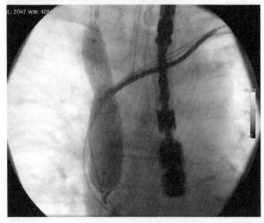

Fig. 3. Fluoroscopy showing inflated occlusion balloon in superior vena cava.

Before usage, several steps need to be taken to ensure successful balloon deployment in the event of a catastrophic complication. A 0.035-inch stiff guidewire must be advanced from the right femoral to the right internal jugular vein. Next, a 12F catheter introducer should be advanced over the stiff guidewire and secured at the insertion site. It is important for the extraction team to rehearse a response protocol if a tear is suspected. This includes preparing a mixture of 12 mL contrast media and 48 mL saline in a Luer Lock syringe. In the event of a possible tear, the balloon is quickly advanced through the sheath and over the stiff guidewire, positioned at the SVC with the guidance of fluoroscopy, connected to the syringe, and inflated.[12]

Experience

SVC tears present one of the most critical complications of transvenous lead extraction. Animal studies have demonstrated just how devastating the associated blood loss is, because a tear sustained for 1 minute correlates with 500 mL of blood loss. Following 10 minutes of an SVC tear, an animal model loses its entire circulating blood volume through exsanguination.[23] Thus, the occlusion balloon was designed to stem this critical blood loss and offer more time and stability for a surgical repair.

The occlusion balloon has been in clinical use since early 2016. Assessment of its early clinical use has demonstrated a statistically significant impact in reducing mortality associated with SVC tears during transvenous lead extraction compared with cases in which the balloon was not used. Furthermore, the balloon is being used prophylactically for patients deemed to be high risk for complications during extractions. For prophylactic use of the balloon, the deflated balloon is placed in either the SVC or inferior vena cava so that, if an injury does occur, it is inflated in a matter of seconds. This would reduce the potential blood loss from a later response time, and a prospective study has demonstrated that prophylactic use in either the SVC or inferior vena cava does not interfere with the extraction and has not been associated with any adverse events.[24] In 2017, a best practice protocol for use of the occlusion balloon was published and its central recommendations are listed in **Box 2**.[25]

SURGICAL REPAIR

Injuries sustained during lead extraction are complex situations where immediate and effective surgical treatment is a clear necessity to prevent mortality. Time is of the essence in the setting of cardiac tamponade because increasing pericardial pressure prevents sufficient cardiac output to maintain neurologic function, and irreversible neurologic injury generally occurs within 5 to 10 minutes. These situations are made even more tenuous because team members, including surgical back-up, may not be familiar with the appropriate management. Even in the setting of rapid balloon deployment, the situation necessitates immediate thoracotomy (usually sternotomy), evacuation of tamponade, and repair of the injury. Simultaneous aggressive maintenance of cardiac output and blood pressure with fluid and vasoconstrictors by the anesthesia team is critical. For large or complex injuries, ongoing blood loss from tears in the right atrium (RA) or SVC may make cardiopulmonary bypass (CPB) and the use of a cardiotomy sucker absolutely necessary because maintenance of cardiac output cannot be achieved otherwise. To be placed on CPB, the patient must be fully anticoagulated with unfractionated heparin, which may seem counterintuitive in the setting of trauma. However, in many cases, maintaining cardiac output and repairing the injury is not achievable without heparinization. Therefore, a CPB pump, and the personnel to operate it, must be immediately available at the location of the extraction because we do not believe it is feasible to transport a patient in this situation (although this strategy has been described). Although smaller injuries may not require CPB, these patients can still quickly develop a large tamponade that often involves clotted and liquid blood. Therefore, pericardiocentesis is only temporarily or partially effective because even if there is a small injury, clotted blood cannot be evacuated by pericardiocentesis.

Despite the severity of some venous and right-sided cardiac tears associated with lead extraction, most are safely repaired, provided that surgical expertise and a CPB pump and perfusionist are immediately available. In the British Columbia series, where intervention was essentially immediate, we found a low mortality (12.1%) given the acuity and magnitude of the injury.[8] Comparative mortalities in recent publications are 27 out of 62 (44%) from the MAUDE database and 36% from another large single-center series at the Cleveland Clinic.[4,20]

Circulatory Collapse

In the setting of circulatory collapse or what we described as a type 1 presentation, the sternum should be opened immediately, and provided that the injury found is indeed moderate to severe, heparin administered, an arterial cannula quickly placed, and preparation made for sucker bypass. Any fashion of venous drainage (including cardiotomy sucker bypass) can be used to restore the circulation, and the inferior vena cava–related lower atrium easily cannulated. Low-pressure but high-volume right heart and central venous bleeding, even when the exact location of the tear cannot be rapidly determined, can usually be controlled with hand or sponge pressure. When the patient is placed on bypass, the right side of the circulation is immediately decompressed, blood loss falls dramatically, and the cardiotomy sucker is used to provide a clear field for the required repair. An umbilical tape around the inferior vena cava cannula, as used in cardiac transplantation or tricuspid valve surgery, is used to prevent air entrapment from the opening in the venous system. Clamping the lower SVC can also prevent air entrapment if the injury is above this area.

Right Ventricular and Right Atrial Appendage Tears

Right ventricular injuries are usually small and easy to control as are RA appendage tears, which are rarely large in size and typically related to removal of the atrial lead (**Fig. 4**). Indeed, in both cases these tears relate to the removal of the electrically active electrode tip where it is fibrosed to the heart. Because of the nature of electrode

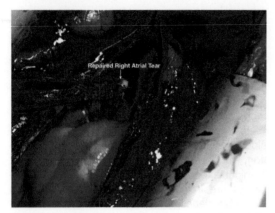

Fig. 4. Intraoperative photograph showing right atrial tear repaired.

placement and the muscularity of the right ventricle, injuries here are usually isolated holes that are easily sutured, and rarely require CPB. A midline subxiphoid incision of 10 to 15 cm was occasionally used in stable patients. With upward traction on the sternum, a good portion of the right ventricle and RA can often be visualized, and tamponade easily evacuated. This is not a suitable incision for SVC injuries but is easily extended into a partial lower sternotomy or full sternotomy should that be necessary.

Superior Vena Cava Injuries

Most studies have found at least half the tears involve the SVC and therefore could be temporized by the occlusion balloon. Although these injuries may involve the proximal innominate or brachiocephalic vein or extend into the RA, the ultracompliant occlusion balloon likely has a benefit in dramatically reducing the blood loss from these injuries. Because of the nature of the SVC, large injuries are much more likely to require a patch repair to maintain patency of this structure.

In addition to an arterial pressure monitoring line, our anesthesia team now places a below-diaphragm large-bore intravenous or central line in every case. The rationale is that injuries often involve the SVC and upper RA. The ability to administer fluid below the diaphragm is helpful if inferior vena cava cannulation (or temporary SVC clamping) is used to isolate the injury, stop bleeding, and restore perfusion using blood returned only from the inferior vena cava. We also pass off a cell-saver suction on every case because this can salvage a large amount of the initial blood loss in case of injury and is inexpensive. Some practitioners have anecdotally advocated the institution of peripheral venoarterial CPB in the setting of these injuries. In our

experience, venoarterial CPB has significant disadvantages. Tamponade prevents venous return to the pump in peripheral venoarterial cannulation, and is significantly more time-consuming to implement. Also, injuries to venous structures can allow for air entrapment and air lock in the open reservoir CPB circuit once the chest is opened.

In the presence of a perforation of the SVC that causes a right hemothorax and no tamponade, a right thoracotomy in the third interspace is a possible approach, although it does not provide for easy institution of CPB. This may also be useful in the setting of previous open-heart surgery where RA and SVC injuries are likely the most common, and opening the sternum is more complicated. Finally, good practices for all institutions that perform lead extraction include:

1. Maintaining a timeout checklist of items that need to be present at the beginning of every extraction (ie, perfusionist, surgeon available, blood available, sternal saw ready).
2. Practice balloon deployment and surgical rescue in a mock code-type situation. This experience is of tremendous value when a true emergency happens.

REFERENCES

1. Candinas R, Duru F, Schneider J, et al. Postmortem analysis of encapsulation around long-term ventricular endocardial pacing leads. Mayo Clin Proc 1999; 74:120–5.
2. Robboy SJ, Harthorne JW, Leinbach RC, et al. Autopsy findings with permanent pervenous pacemakers. Circulation 1969;39:495–501.
3. Bracke F, Meijer A, Van Gelder B. Extraction of pacemaker and implantable cardioverter defibrillator leads. Pacing Clin Electrophysiol 2002;25(7): 1037–40.
4. Hauser RG, Katsiyiannis WT, Gornick CC, et al. Deaths and cardiovascular injuries due to device-assisted implantable cardioverter-defibrillator and pacemaker lead extraction. Europace 2010;12(3): 395–401.
5. Jones SO, Eckart RE, Albert CM, et al. Large single-center, single-operator experience with transvenous lead extraction: outcomes and changing indications. Heart Rhythm 2008;5(4):520–5.
6. Brunner MP, Cronin EM, Wazni O, et al. Outcomes of patients requiring emergent surgical or endovascular intervention for catastrophic complications during transvenous lead extraction. Heart Rhythm 2014;11:419–25.
7. Wazni O, Epstein LM, Carrillo RG, et al. Lead extraction in the contemporary setting: the LExICon study. An observational retrospective study of consecutive

laser lead extractions. J Am Coll Cardiol 2010;55: 579–86.

8. Bashir J, Fedoruk LM, O'fiesh J, et al. Classification and surgical repair of injuries sustained during transvenous lead extraction. Circ Arrhythm Electrophysiol 2016;9 [pii:e003741].

9. Wang W, Wang X, Modry D, et al. Cardiopulmonary bypass standby avoids fatality due to vascular laceration in laser-assisted lead extraction. J Card Surg 2014;29:274–8.

10. Agarwal SK, Kamireddy S, Nemec J, et al. Predictors of complications of endovascular chronic lead extractions from pacemakers and defibrillators: a single center experience. J Cardiovasc Electrophysiol 2009;20:171–5.

11. Kennergren C, Bucknall CA, Butter C, et al. Laser assisted lead extraction: the European experience. Europace 2007;9:651–6.

12. Azarrafiy R, Tsang DC, Boyle TA, et al. Compliant endovascular balloon reduces the lethality of superior vena cava tears during transvenous lead extractions. Heart Rhythm 2017;14(9):1400–4.

13. Holinski S, Jessen S, Neumann K, et al. Predictive power and implication of Euroscore, Euroscore II and STS Score for isolated repeat aortic valve replacement. Ann Thorac Cardiovasc Surg 2015; 21:242–6.

14. Ad N, Barnett SD, Speir AM. Performance of the Euroscore and the Society of Thoracic Surgeons mortality risk score: the gender factor. Interact Cardiovasc Thorac Surg 2007;6:192–5.

15. Kusumoto FM, Schoenfeld MH, Wilkoff B, et al. 2017 HRS expert consensus statement on cardiovascular implantable electronic device lead management and extraction. Heart Rhythm 2017; 14(12). E503–e551.

16. Byrd CL, Wilkoff BL, Love CJ, et al. Intravascular extraction of problematic or infected permanent pacemaker leads. Pacing Clin Electrophysiol 1999; 22:1348–57.

17. Byrd CL, Wilkoff BL, Love CJ, et al. Clinical study of the laser sheath for lead extraction: the total experience in the United States. Pacing Clin Electrophysiol 2002;25:804–8.

18. Bongiorni MG, Kennergren C, Butter C, et al. The European lead extraction controlled study. A European Heart Rhythm Association registry of transvenous lead extraction outcomes. Eur Heart J 2017; 38:2995–3005.

19. Epstein LM, Love CJ, Wilkoff BL, et al. Superior vena cava defibrillator coils make transvenous lead extraction more challenging and riskier. J Am Coll Cardiol 2013;61:987–8.

20. Brunner MP, Cronin EM, Duarte VE, et al. Clinical predictors of adverse patient outcomes in an experience of more than 5000 chronic endovascular pacemaker and defibrillator lead extractions. Heart Rhythm 2014;11:799–805.

21. Bordacher P, Defaye P, Peyrouse E, et al. Extraction of old pacemaker and cardioverter-defibrillator leads by laser sheath vs femoral approach. Circ Arrhythm Electrophysiol 2010;3:319–23.

22. Caniglia-Miller JM, Bussey WD, Kamtz NM, et al. Surgical management of major intrathoracic hemorrhage resulting from high-risk transvenous pacemaker/defibrillator lead extraction. J Card Surg 2015;30:149–53.

23. Clancy JF, Carrillo RG, Sotak R, et al. Percutaneous occlusion balloon as a bridge to surgery in a swine model of superior vena cava perforation. Heart Rhythm 2016;13(11):2215–20.

24. Tsang DC, Azarrafiy R, Pecha S, et al. Long-term outcomes of prophylactic placement of an endovascular balloon in the vena cava for high-risk transvenous lead extractions. Heart Rhythm 2017;14(12):1833–8.

25. Wilkoff BL, Kennergren C, Love CJ, et al. Bridge to surgery: best practice protocol derived from early clinical experience with the bridge occlusion balloon. Federated agreement from the eleventh annual lead management symposium. Heart Rhythm 2017;14(10):1574–8.

Surgical and Hybrid Lead Extraction

Ryan Azarrafiy, BA[a], Roger G. Carrillo, MD, MBA, FHRS[b],*

KEYWORDS

- Lead extraction • Surgery • Minimally invasive • Transvenous • Hybrid
- Cardiac implantable electronic device • Pacemaker • Implantable cardioverter-defibrillator

KEY POINTS

- Several minimally invasive surgical approaches serve as alternatives to median sternotomy for lead extractions that are unamenable to standard, percutaneous approaches.
- The transatrial, subxiphoid, left minithoracotomy/thoracoscopy, and ministernotomy are 4 minimally invasive procedures for lead extractions in which a percutaneous approach is unfeasible.
- A hybrid open heart surgery and transvenous lead extraction can be performed for patients with infected or malfunctioning devices who present with concomitant conditions such as valvulopathies or coronary artery disease.
- A multidisciplinary decision-making process involving cardiac electrophysiologists, cardiac surgeons, radiologists, and anesthesiologists is critical to ensuring safe and effective lead extractions for standard and complex cases.

INTRODUCTION

Cardiac implantable electronic devices are a cornerstone of medical practice; millions of patients worldwide have cardiac arrhythmias requiring treatment with these devices.[1] Yet, in rare circumstances, cardiac implantable electronic devices can become infected or malfunction. In these cases, removal of both the device generator and its associated leads is indicated. In a procedure called lead extraction, device leads implanted for more than 1 year are removed with specialized equipment, often through the transvenous use of a laser-powered sheath. Lead extraction has been proven to be a safe and effective procedure that is performed almost exclusively through a percutaneous approach. In this procedure, cardiac electrophysiologists choose to perform the extraction through the subclavian vein or, in more complex cases, through the femoral vein.[2] However, certain complex cases may not be amenable to either of these percutaneous techniques, and require a surgical approach. Although the traditional approach to complex cases not amenable to percutaneous extraction has been a median sternotomy and open removal of device and leads, several minimally invasive methods have been developed and used, offering a range of alternatives to a full open heart procedure with sternotomy.

Some patients, however, may present with concomitant conditions such as coronary artery disease or valvulopathies in addition to an infected or malfunctioning cardiac implantable electronic device. These cases are treated with a hybrid approach, which we define as open heart surgery and transvenous lead extraction (TLE) in a single, combined procedure. Thus, the role of surgery in

Disclosure: R. Azarrafiy has no disclosures. R.G. Carrillo has served as a consultant to Spectranetics and Sensormatic; has received a research grant from St. Jude Medical; and has served on the Speakers Bureau for Medtronic, St. Jude Medical, and the Sorin Group.
Funding: No funding was received for the writing of this article.
^a University of Miami Miller School of Medicine, Miami, FL, USA; ^b The Heart Institute at Palmetto General Hospital, 7150 West 20th Avenue, Suite 615, Hialeah, FL 33016, USA
* Corresponding author.
E-mail address: rogercar@aol.com

cardiacEP.theclinics.com

lead extraction falls under 2 categories: surgical lead extraction without any concomitant conditions and hybrid open heart surgery and TLE for concomitant conditions (**Fig. 1**).

In this article, we explain and assess our institution's experience with 4 minimally invasive surgical approaches to lead extraction. Furthermore, we describe our experience with hybrid procedures for patients who present with concomitant conditions.

MINIMALLY INVASIVE SURGICAL LEAD EXTRACTION

The standard approach for a cardiac device lead extraction is a percutaneous procedure, through either the subclavian or femoral vein. If these procedures fail or are contraindicated, the traditional next step has been to perform a median sternotomy and open removal of the leads and device. However, 4 surgical approaches offer a less invasive alternative to an open extraction. These approaches include the transatrial approach, the subxiphoid approach, the left minithoracotomy/thoracoscopy, and the ministernotomy.

The Transatrial Approach

The transatrial approach involves a minimally invasive incision to remove the leads directly from the right atrium under fluoroscopic guidance. This procedure offers an alternative to median sternotomy for leads that have perforated the right atrium or lead fragments that have been abandoned and could not be retrieved by conventional, transvenous techniques.

Technique

In the transatrial approach, the patient is placed under general anesthesia. The patient is intubated with a single lumen endotracheal tube including a right bronchial blocker. An arterial line is obtained for blood pressure and large venous lines are placed for volume resuscitation. The patient is placed in the supine position. A small, 2-inch incision is made at the level of the fourth intercostal space from the midclavicular line to the anterior axillary line. The ribs and pleura are dissected, and a longitudinal 2-inch incision is used to open the pericardium anterior to the phrenic nerve. A purse string is placed on the right atrium. The lung is collapsed and under fluoroscopic guidance, the lead is retrieved and pulled out of the right atrium using a rongeur. Laser or mechanical tools are used to remove the leads from the heart in an antegrade or retrograde direction. The extraction sheath is advanced in the direction of either the apex of the heart or the subclavian vein, depending on the segment that must be removed. The whole procedure can be done with or without the aid of an endoscope. The actual extraction process is guided with fluoroscopy (**Fig. 2**). After the extraction, an 18F chest tube is placed and removed 24 hours after the procedure.

Authors' experience

At our center, 14 cases used a transatrial approach between January 2003 and October

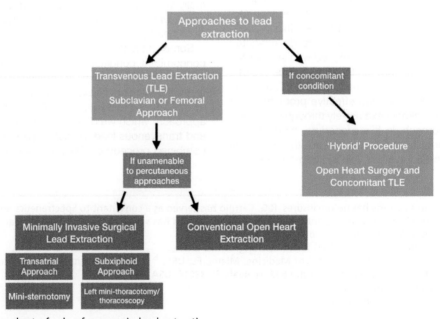

Fig. 1. Flow chart of role of surgery in lead extraction.

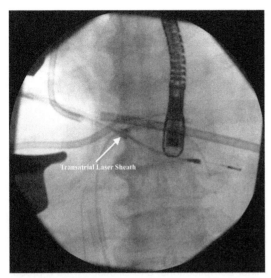

Fig. 2. Fluoroscopic image of lead extraction through a transatrial approach.

2017 (**Table 1**). The average age for patients undergoing the procedure was 64.14 ± 20.9 years. Eleven patient were male (78.6%)and 3 were female (21.4%). The devices extracted were as follows: 8 pacemakers (57.2%), 5 implantable cardioverter-defibrillators (ICDs; 35.7%), and 1 cardiac resynchronization therapy defibrillator (CRTD; 7.1%). The average lead dwell time was 10.5 ± 6.96 years. Eleven devices were extracted owing to infection (78.6%) and the remaining devices were extracted owing to malfunction (21.4%). Of the 14 cases that used the transatrial

approach, there were no major complications and 1 minor hematoma. All cases were a procedural success and all patients were discharged alive.

The Subxiphoid Approach

The subxiphoid approach involves an incision inferior to the xiphoid process to extract leads that have chronically perforated the right ventricle or the vestibule of the right atrium. Furthermore, this technique is used to extract epicardial leads.

Technique

In the subxiphoid approach, the patient is placed under general anesthesia. The patient is intubated with a single lumen endotracheal tube. An arterial line is obtained for blood pressure and large venous lines are placed for volume resuscitation. The patient is placed in supine position. A 2-inch incision is made just inferior to the xiphoid process and a retractor is used to lift the sternum upward. The pericardium is opened and the leads are visualized. The leads may be extracardiac or epicardial. If they are extracardiac, the protruding portion may be removed from the subxiphoid approach. First, a purse string is placed and then the distal end of the lead is cut at the level of the myocardium. The lead will retract into the ventricle. The purse string is tied, and the more proximal portions of the lead can then be removed through a standard percutaneous approach. For epicardial leads, dissection with electrocautery at a low voltage setting can be helpful and at times

Table 1
Case information and demographics for minimally invasive procedures

Approach	Transatrial (n = 14)	Subxiphoid (n = 11)	Left Minithoracotomy (n = 19)	Ministernotomy (n = 1)
Age, mean ± SD	64.14 ± 20.9	62.5 ± 16.6	66.2 ± 14.3	59
Sex	3 Female (21.4) 11 Male (78.6)	3 Female (27.3) 8 Male (72.7)	5 Female (26.3) 14 Male (73.7)	Male
Device extracted	5 ICD (35.7) 8 PPM (57.2) 1 CRTD (7.1)	2 ICD (18.2) 3 PPM (27.3) 6 CRTD (54.5)	8 ICD (42.1) 4 PPM (21.1) 7 CRTD (36.8)	ICD
Lead dwell time (y)	10.5 (±6.96)	10.1 (±10.3)	7.15 (±6.52)	7.8
Indication	11 Infection (78.6) 3 Malfunction (21.4)	9 Infection (81.8) 2 Malfunction (18.2)	13 Infection (68.4) 6 Malfunction (31.6)	Infection
Major complication	0 (0.0)	0 (0.0)	0 (0.0)	No
Minor complication	1 Hematoma (7.1)	0 (0.0)	0 (0.0)	No
Procedural success	14 (100.0)	11 (100.0)	19 (100.0)	Yes
Survival at discharge	14 (100.0)	10 (90.9)	18 (94.7)	Yes

Abbreviations: AVR CRTD, cardiac resynchronization therapy defibrillator; ICD, implantable cardioverter-defibrillator; PPM, permanent pacemaker; SD, standard deviation.

may be assisted by fluoroscopy. After lead removal, hemostasis is obtained, a 10-mm flat drain is placed in the pericardial space before skin closure, and the small incision is closed. The drain is removed 24 hours after the procedure.

Authors' experience

Our center has performed a total of 11 subxiphoid extractions from January 2003 to October 2017 (see **Table 1**). The average age of these patients was 62.5 ± 16.6 years. Eight patients were male (72.7%) and 3 were female (27.3%). Six extracted devices were CRTDs (54.5%), 3 devices were pacemakers (27.3%), and 2 devices were ICDs (18.2%). In all cases, the patient had epicardial leads. The average lead dwell time was 10.1 ± 10.3 years. Nine cases required extraction owing to infection (81.8%) and 2 extractions were due to device malfunction (18.2%). There were no major or minor complications, and all cases were a procedural success. Survival at discharge was 90.9% because there was 1 death owing to sepsis unrelated to the procedure.

The Left Minithoracotomy/Thoracoscopy

If there is an extracardiac lead located more toward the apex or left side of the heart, the left minithoracotomy or thoracoscopy can be used. Moreover, this approach can be used for leads that have perforated the coronary sinus or leads located in the epicardium of the left ventricle.

Technique

In the left minithoracotomy/thoracoscopy approach, the patient is placed under general anesthesia. The patient is intubated with a single lumen endotracheal tube and a left bronchial blocker could be used to collapse the lung. An arterial line is obtained for blood pressure and large venous lines are placed for volume resuscitation. Fluoroscopy is first used to locate the exact location of leads to determine where an incision is to be made. Next, a small incision is made in an intercostal space that varies based on the exact location of leads that was determined by fluoroscopy. The ribs, pleura, and pericardium are dissected anterior to the phrenic nerve. If the lead has perforated the coronary sinus, the protruding portion may be removed using the left minithoracotomy/thoracoscopy approach. First, a purse string is placed and then the distal end of the lead is cut at the level of the myocardium. The lead will retract into the ventricle. The purse string is tied and the more proximal portions of the lead can then be removed through a standard percutaneous approach. If the lead being extracted is epicardial, an endoscope can be used to guide the dissection process with electrocautery at a low-voltage setting (**Fig. 3**). An 18F chest tube is placed before skin closure and removed 24 hours after the procedure.

Authors' experience

Our institution has performed 19 left minithoracotomies or thoracoscopies between January 2003 and October 2017 (see **Table 1**). The average age of these patients was 66.2 ± 14.3 years. Fourteen patients were male (73.7%) and 5 were female (26.3%). Eight extracted devices were ICDs (42.1%), 7 were CRTDs (36.8%), and 4 were pacemakers (21.1%). The average lead dwell time was 7.15 ± 6.52 years. Thirteen extractions were due to infection (68.4%) and 6 were due to malfunction (31.6%). Fourteen cases involved extraction of epicardial leads (73.7%). There were no major or minor complications, and all cases were a procedural success. Survival at discharge was 94.7%; there was 1 death owing to ventricular tachycardia in the postoperative period.

The Ministernotomy

The ministernotomy is a rare procedure for patients with retained lead segments in the innominate vein that could not be removed through other methods.

Technique

In the ministernotomy, the patient is placed under general anesthesia. The patient is intubated with a single lumen endotracheal tube. An arterial line is obtained for blood pressure and large venous lines are placed for volume resuscitation. In this procedure, the lead fragment is located under fluoroscopy. The manubrium is then cut from the jugular notch up to the second intercostal space with a small, sternal saw. A retractor is used to open the manubrium. Proximal and distal control of the

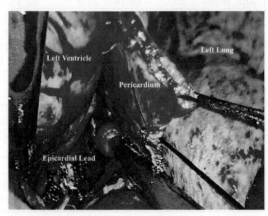

Fig. 3. Endoscopic view of epicardial lead extraction through a left thoracoscopy approach.

innominate vein is obtained. The vein is then opened, the fragment is removed, and a direct or patch repair is performed to close the vein. The sternum is reapproximated with a single stainless steel wire. The skin is closed without drainage.

Case example

This procedure has been performed once at our institution. The case involved a 59-year-old man with sepsis and nonischemic, dilated cardiomyopathy who had previously undergone failed TLEs at different institutions. Despite numerous attempts at a percutaneous approach, an infected ICD lead fragment was retained in the left innominate vein (**Fig. 4**). The lead dwell time for the fragment was 7.8 years. The patient was referred to our center for surgical management. Owing to the prior failed extractions, a decision was made for the patient to undergo a ministernotomy. The procedure was successful and a subcutaneous ICD was placed 1 week after the extraction. The patient was discharged with no complications 12 days after the original procedure.

OPEN HEART SURGERY AND CONCOMITANT TRANSVENOUS LEAD EXTRACTION

At times, patients present with concomitant conditions necessitating a hybrid approach. These conditions may include tricuspid valve endocarditis or valve stenosis. In these cases, a median sternotomy is performed to treat the concomitant condition. Furthermore, the right atrium is opened under cardiopulmonary bypass and the distal end of leads are cut and removed. Then, laser or mechanical tools are used to remove the proximal lead fragments through a percutaneous approach (**Fig. 5**).

At our center, 28 cases involved a concomitant open heart procedure and TLE (**Table 2**). The

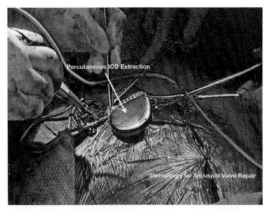

Fig. 5. Percutaneous lead extraction after tricuspid valve repair in a hybrid procedure.

mean age of patients undergoing a combined procedure was 70.75 ± 11.6 years. Twenty-one patients were male (75.0%) and 7 were female (25.0%). Eleven extracted devices were pacemakers (39.3%), 11 were ICDs (39.3%), and 6 were CRTDs (21.4%). The average lead dwell time was 7.97 ± 8.36 years. The most common surgical repairs in the combined procedure were a mitral valve repair (32.1%) and coronary artery bypass grafting with a mitral valve repair (32.1%). Aortic valve replacements, atrial septal defect repairs, and tricuspid valve repairs were also performed. Many of these procedures also involved the removal of large vegetations attached to device leads and heart valves. Of the 28 cases involving a combined procedure, 26 cases (92.9%) resulted in procedural success and survival at discharge. One death was due to pulmonary embolism and the other was due to coagulopathy from advanced cardiac cirrhosis.

DISCUSSION

Surgical lead extraction has evolved significantly over the past several decades. In 1981, Choo and colleagues[3] reported the open extraction of infected epicardial pacemaker systems. Furthermore, in 1998 Varma and colleagues[4] reported a staged extraction involving a percutaneous laser and open surgical approach to extract a chronic atrial lead. In 2010, Rusanov and Spotnitz[5] reported a 15-year experience in which epicardial leads and patches were removed through a median sternotomy or a left, right, or subxiphoid thoracotomy. More recently, institutions have begun to describe minimally invasive surgical approaches to extract leads as an alternative to median sternotomy or full left or right thoracotomies. For example, in 2012 Curnis and colleagues[6]

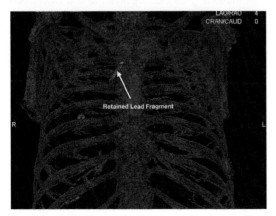

Fig. 4. Three-dimensional reconstruction of a computed tomography imaging showing retained lead fragment in the left innominate vein.

Table 2
Case information and demographics for concomitant procedures

Variables	Means and Frequencies (n = 28)
Age	70.75 ± 11.6
Sex	7 Female (25.0)
	21 Male (75.0)
Device extracted	6 CRTD (21.4)
	11 ICD (39.3)
	11 PPM (39.3)
Combined surgical repair	1 AVR (3.6)
	2 CABG (7.1)
	1 CABG and AVR (3.6)
	9 CABG and MVR (32.1)
	1 CABG and MVR and ASD repair (3.6)
	1 CABG and TVR (3.6)
	9 MVR (32.1)
	1 MVR and TVR (3.6)
	3 TVR (10.7)
Lead dwell time (y)	7.97 ± 8.36
Major complication	2 (7.1)
Minor complication	3 (10.7)
Procedural success	26 (92.9)
Survival at discharge	26 (92.9)

Abbreviations: ASD, atrial septal defect; AVR, aortic valve replacement; CABG, coronary artery bypass graft; CRTD, cardiac resynchronization therapy defibrillator; ICD, implantable cardioverter-defibrillator; MVR, mitral valve repair; PPM, permanent pacemaker; SD, standard deviation; TVR, tricuspid valve repair.

described using a left thoracoscopy to complete a failed percutaneous coronary sinus lead extraction. Several institutions have also described the use of the right minithoracotomy, which we have described as the "transatrial" approach, to extract fractured leads or those unamenable to a percutaneous extraction.[7–10] Overall, surgical extraction has advanced significantly over the past several decades with minimally invasive approaches serving as safe and effective alternatives to median sternotomy in cases unamenable to percutaneous extraction.

The role of the cardiac surgeon has also changed in the dynamic field of lead extraction. Before the advent of mechanical and laser tools to percutaneously remove devices, surgery was the only option for patients. Although cardiac surgeons continue to play a significant role in both the implantation and extraction of epicardial leads, lead extraction today is done almost exclusively through a percutaneous approach.[2] Yet, as the literature and our center's experience have shown, the cardiac surgeon can

play a critical role in using minimally invasive techniques to extract leads in which a percutaneous approach is not feasible. In addition to this extraction option, the cardiac surgeon also serves as an essential backup response in the inevitable event of complications. For example, Bernardes de Souza and colleagues[11] report a series of three cases involving vascular injury in which an urgent surgical response prevented mortality. Overall, multiple single center studies and expert guidelines report that a multidisciplinary approach to lead extraction involving electrophysiologists and cardiac surgeons ensures both safe and successful procedures.[11–13]

Another significant role for cardiac surgery in lead extraction is for patients who present with concomitant conditions necessitating both open heart surgery and TLE. At our center, we describe performing these procedures in a single, combined procedure, which we define as a hybrid procedure. However, it is important to note that this definition of hybrid is different from how the term has been used by other centers. Other institutions describe hybrid procedures as those in which a cardiac surgeon performs the incision for a minimally invasive extraction, and electrophysiologists then use a laser or mechanical sheath to remove the lead.[7] At our center, the clinician performing lead extractions is also a cardiac surgeon, so these procedures are simply termed minimally invasive surgical extractions and are performed entirely by a single operator. We use the term hybrid for cases in which open heart surgery is needed in addition to TLE for a concomitant condition. Thus, these hybrid procedures present another unique role for the cardiac surgeon in lead extraction.

Overall, several tools and approaches can be used to safely and effectively manage infected or malfunctioning cardiac devices, and a multidisciplinary decision-making process is critical to a successful procedure. The standard approach to lead extraction is a percutaneous approach through the subclavian vein with the use of laser or mechanical tools. However, certain extractions cannot be accomplished through a subclavian route. Alternative percutaneous methods have been successfully described including a femoral or internal jugular approach as well as a combined approach of the two.[14] However, certain cases are still not amenable to these percutaneous alternatives, requiring a surgical approach. In the planning stage of lead extraction, a thorough radiologic analysis can help to determine if leads are extracardiac or abandoned. In these cases, a multidisciplinary conversation between cardiac electrophysiologists, cardiac surgeons, radiologists, and cardiac anesthesiologists can help to identify cases in which a minimally invasive, surgical lead extraction may be necessary. These procedures should be performed by an operator with significant experience in the surgical management of device leads. In the case of concomitant conditions, electrophysiologists and cardiac surgeons may need to coordinate to perform an open heart procedure and TLE in a single, combined procedure.

SUMMARY

Several surgical options exist for cases not amenable to conventional, percutaneous approaches to lead extraction. At our institution, the transatrial approach, the subxiphoid approach, the left minithoracotomy/thoracoscopy, and the ministernotomy are minimally invasive, surgical approaches that have been safe and effective alternatives to median sternotomy in complex cases. These approaches may be considered by cardiac surgeons involved in lead extraction. Furthermore, hybrid extraction is a consideration in patients who present with concomitant conditions requiring cardiac surgery such as coronary artery disease or valve endocarditis. Open heart surgery and TLE have been successfully performed as a combined procedure at our institution and is a feasible approach for treatment of patients with associated pathologies.

REFERENCES

1. Zhan C, Baine WB, Sedrakyan A, et al. Cardiac device implantation in the United States from 1997 through 2004: a population-based analysis. J Gen Intern Med 2008;23(Suppl 1):13–9.
2. Kusumoto FM, Schoenfeld MH, Wilkoff BL, et al. HRS expert consensus statement on cardiovascular implantable electronic device lead management and extraction. Heart Rhythm 2017;14(12):e503–51.
3. Choo MH, Holmes DR Jr, Gersh BJ, et al. Infected epicardial pacemaker systems. Partial versus total removal. J Thorac Cardiovasc Surg 1981;82(5): 794–6.
4. Varma NJ, Sellke FW, Epstein LM. Chronic atrial lead explantation using a staged percutaneous laser and open surgical approach. Pacing Clin Electrophysiol 1998;21(7):1483–5.
5. Rusanov A, Spotnitz HM. A 15-year experience with permanent pacemaker and defibrillator lead and patch extractions. Ann Thorac Surg 2010;89(1): 44–50.
6. Curnis A, Bontempi L, Coppola G, et al. Active-fixation coronary sinus pacing lead extraction: a hybrid approach. Int J Cardiol 2012;156(3):e51–2.
7. Bontempi L, Vassanelli F, Cerini M, et al. Hybrid minimally invasive approach for transvenous lead extraction: a feasible technique in high-risk patients. J Cardiovasc Electrophysiol 2017;28(4):466–73.
8. Goyal SK, Ellis CR, Ball SK, et al. High-risk lead removal by planned sequential transvenous laser extraction and minimally invasive right thoracotomy. J Cardiovasc Electrophysiol 2014;25(6):617–21.
9. Koneru JN, Ellenbogen KA. High-risk lead extraction using a hybrid approach: the blade and the light-saber. J Cardiovasc Electrophysiol 2014;25(6): 622–3.
10. Rodriguez Y, Garisto JD, Carrillo RG. A novel retrograde laser extraction technique using a transatrial approach: an alternative for complex lead extractions. Circ Arrhythm Electrophysiol 2011;4(4):501–5.
11. Bernardes de Souza B, Benharash P, Esmailian F, et al. Value of a joint cardiac surgery-cardiac electrophysiology approach to lead extraction. J Card Surg 2015;30(11):874–6.
12. Maus TM, Shurter J, Nguyen L, et al. Multidisciplinary approach to transvenous lead extraction: a single center's experience. J Cardiothorac Vasc Anesth 2015;29(2):265–70.
13. Wilkoff BL, Love CJ, Byrd CL, et al. Transvenous lead extraction: heart rhythm society expert consensus on facilities, training, indications, and patient management: this document was endorsed by the American Heart Association (AHA). Heart Rhythm 2009;6(7):1085–104.
14. Mulpuru SK, Hayes DL, Osborn MJ, et al. Femoral approach to lead extraction. J Cardiovasc Electrophysiol 2015;26(3):357–61.

Patient Management

Reimplantation After Lead Removal

Mohamed B. Elshazly, MD[a], Khaldoun G. Tarakji, MD, MPH[b],*

KEYWORDS

• CIED • Extraction • Reimplantation • Pacemaker • Defibrillator • Leads

KEY POINTS

- The number of implanted cardiovascular implantable electronic devices (CIEDs) has increased significantly in the last 30 years.
- This increase has led to an upsurge in CIED complications, such as infection and lead malfunction requiring CIED extraction.
- Following extraction, the decision-making process of CIED reimplantation requires meticulous planning that includes careful consideration of several aspects, including the reason for extraction, the indication for CIED reimplantation, patients' wishes, timing of reimplantation, the need for a bridging device, and the type and location of device to be reimplanted.
- In this article, the authors review this decision-making process and the necessary steps to achieve optimal patient outcomes.

INTRODUCTION

Over the last 6 decades, cardiovascular implantable electronic devices (CIEDs), including permanent pacemakers, implantable cardioverter-defibrillators (ICDs), and cardiac resynchronization therapy (CRT-D [with defibrillator] and CRT-P [without defibrillator]), have become a cornerstone in the management of patients with heart rhythm disorders and heart failure as well as the prevention of sudden cardiac death. It is estimated that 1.2 to 1.4 million CIEDs are currently implanted annually around the world.[1] As the number of implanted CIEDs increases and as patients live longer requiring multiple pulse generator changes, system upgrades, or lead revisions, we will continue to witness an increasing rate of device-related complications, such as infection and device malfunction, requiring extraction. The rate of CIED infection has been estimated at 0.5% with primary implants and 1.0% to 7.0% with secondary interventions,[2]

although incidence reports have varied widely. Moreover, the rate of increase in CIED infection is outpacing the rate of increase in CIED implantation; one study showed a 12% increase in the number of CIED implantations from 2004 to 2006, with a 57% increment in CIED infections during the same period.[3] Another study showed there was a sharp increase in the number of CIED infections after 2004 coinciding with an increase in comorbidities within patients undergoing implantation.[4] In addition to infection, the rate of device malfunction still occurs at a higher-than-desired rate with a 5-year failure rate of ICD leads of 2.5% per one report.[5] The relatively high rate of device malfunction and the upsurge in device-related infections has led to a corresponding increase in the number of extraction procedures performed, which come with their own set of procedural complications.

The first stage of management of patients with CIED infection or malfunction is extraction; yet, the second stage of reimplantation is equally

Disclosures: M.B. Elshazly: none. K.G. Tarakji: advisory board/consulting: Medtronic, AliveCor.
[a] Division of Cardiology, Department of Medicine, Weill Cornell Medical College, Doha, Qatar; [b] Department of Cardiac Electrophysiology and Pacing, Heart and Vascular Institute, Cleveland Clinic, 9500 Euclid Avenue J2-2, Cleveland, OH 44195, USA
* Corresponding author.
E-mail address: tarakjk@ccf.org

Card Electrophysiol Clin 10 (2018) 667–674
https://doi.org/10.1016/j.ccep.2018.04.004

important to take into consideration, and planning the strategy for reimplantation should occur simultaneously with planning for extraction. Reimplantation consideration starts with some basic and fundamental questions. Is the CIED still indicated? And if so, is it needed during the same procedure or same hospitalization? In observational studies, one-third of patients did not require their CIED reimplanted during the same hospitalization after undergoing extraction for CIED infection.[6,7] This finding was due to the change in clinical status of the patients, the ability to delay the procedure to achieve other clinical or social goals, or the lack of a clear initial indication for device implantation. In another case series of patients who underwent extraction for various indications, 14% did not undergo reimplantation mostly because they no longer met CIED indications. These patients had higher mortality, compared with those who underwent reimplantation, because of their higher comorbidities and not because of arrhythmic events.[8] Given the potential for significant complications and cost linked to CIED implantation and extraction procedures, it is absolutely necessary that cardiac electrophysiologists corroborate the patients' indication for CIED implantation and make sure that implantation is performed in an optimal and minimal-risk setting. In this article, the authors aim to review reimplantation after lead removal and answer the following questions: How is reimplantation different after extraction of infected versus noninfected leads? When is the optimal time to reimplant and where? Should there be a bridge to reimplantation? What kind of device should be reimplanted to avoid future complications?

DECISION-MAKING PROCESS FOR REIMPLANTATION
Reimplantation After Extraction of Noninfected Cardiovascular Implantable Electronic Device

Recent advances in extraction tools, such as the use of laser sheaths, powered mechanical sheaths, superior vena cava (SVC)–compliant occlusive rescue balloons, and hybrid operating rooms at high-volume centers, have led to an increase in the safety and volume of successful CIED extractions performed. Although extracting infected leads is the standard of care, there has been a debate about whether we should be extracting versus abandoning and capping noninfected ones. This question comes up when patients are undergoing a system upgrade (eg, upgrading a pacemaker to defibrillator) or when there is lead malfunction.[5] Two recent studies

have shed some light on this debate. In one study of patients with noninfected lead failure, Pokorney and colleagues[9] examined a Medicare sample of 6859 patients who had leads abandoned and capped (N = 5746, 83.8%) or extracted (N = 1113) 12 months or more after the de novo implantation. Over a median follow-up of 2.4 years, elective lead extraction for noninfectious indications had similar long-term survival to that for abandoning and capping leads; however, extraction was associated with a lower risk of device infection at 5 years. A recent case series at the Cleveland Clinic showed that noninfected transvenous lead extraction (719 leads) at the time of system upgrade was associated with a low complication rate, with a 97% clinical success rate.[10]

The common practice of abandoning leads mitigates acute extraction procedural complications yet can potentially lead to long-term complications, such as vascular access patency, tricuspid valvular regurgitation, possible increase in long-term infection risk, and most importantly increasing the complexity of future necessary extraction of infected leads. A recent analysis from the authors' institution of 1386 patients with infected CIEDs showed that 23% had previously abandoned leads. Failure to achieve complete procedural success without major complications was 4-fold higher in those with existing abandoned leads. Moreover, abandoned leads were associated with a higher rate of retained lead material, longer procedural and fluoroscopy times, and increased use of specialized extraction tools, such as femoral workstation.[11] These data suggest that, at high-volume centers with low complication rates, extraction of noninfected failed leads or extraction at the time of system upgrade should be at least considered and discussed with patients in order to avoid potential long-term complications associated with having multiple abandoned leads. This point is particularly relevant in younger patients with relatively newer leads. Multidisciplinary discussion between the cardiac electrophysiologist, anesthesiologist, and backup cardiac surgeon is necessary to determine the patients' risk of procedural complications and the risk of open heart surgery if needed. The short- and long-term complications of extracting versus abandoning leads should then be discussed with the patients in a well-informed shared decision-making process.

Before noninfected lead extraction and reimplantation, the operator must plan the procedure meticulously and take specific technical factors into consideration. It is always recommended to secure a new venous access before performing lead extraction to guarantee the ability to reimplant if needed. If the extracted lead failed because of access being too medial or too lateral and mechanical stresses, every effort should be made to provide a less stressful access for the new lead. When new venous access is not possible, then the following strategies should be taken into account. In most cases, the new lead is reimplanted on the same side as the extracted lead. Thus, it is crucial that the operator maintains adequate venous access after lead extraction, which depends on the degree of lead adhesion onto the venous wall. Old leads, usually greater than 5 years old, are likely to have strong adhesions,[12] thus, allowing the operator to advance the extraction sheath over the lead creating a track needed to subsequently advance a wire and secure access for the introducer sheath and new lead. The introducer sheath should be long enough to reach the right atrium avoiding potential complications, as there may be stenosis of the access vein and potential weakening of the vessel walls secondary to the extraction. However, a relatively recent lead may be weakly adhered to the venous wall, thus, it can slide out easily while advancing the extraction sheath over it. In the scenario with a young lead, the operator should be prepared to snare the lead tip from the inferior vena cava using femoral venous access and a snare, such as a gooseneck snare. This technique provides tensile support for advancing the extraction sheath over the lead, thus, creating the route necessary to subsequently place the new lead. Another issue the operator should consider during reimplantation is the site of fixation for the new lead. In many instances, the old lead tip is extracted along with a small piece of myocardial tissue. Screwing the new lead in the same exact site may increase the chance of perforation. Moreover, this area may be fibrosed with damaged myocardial tissue leading to increased capture thresholds and inadequate sensing. The operator must take these factors into consideration and consider implanting the new lead in a different myocardial site.

Reimplantation After Extraction of Infected Cardiovascular Implantable Electronic Device

CIED infection is a highly morbid condition with high morbidity and mortality at 1 year even after device extraction.[13] CIED extraction is a class I indication for infection. Extraction procedures offer a renewed opportunity to reassess the indications for CIED reimplantation. Some patients may have had interval improvement in their rhythm or ejection fraction (EF) with resultant resolution of the initial indication to place a CIED. Moreover, some patients may prefer not to receive a new CIED when significant comorbidities and high short-term mortality outweigh the benefit. In some other cases, the CIED may have been implanted for a relative rather than absolute indication, such as chronotropic incompetence. In such cases, reimplanting a device after a device-related infection may carry more harm than benefit for patients. Finally, some patients refuse to have a new CIED implanted and their wishes must be respected. The decision to reimplant a CIED is a shared process between patients and their cardiologist. It is imperative that such a discussion takes place before device extraction and should be reaffirmed once patients are ready for reimplantation.

The authors review some common scenarios whereby reimplantation may not be indicated. First, a 65-year-old man with a history of nonischemic cardiomyopathy with an EF of 32% and primary prevention single chamber ICD implanted 10 years ago presents with pocket infection complicated by vegetations on the lead and systemic bacteremia. In the last 10 years, he had no ventricular arrhythmia events and no tachyarrhythmia therapies delivered. His most recent echocardiogram revealed an EF of 50%. It was recommended he undergo full CIED extraction for his current endocarditis, and he is questioning whether he needs to have a new primary prevention ICD reimplanted. Although the patient has no absolute indication to place a new ICD given the improvement of EF to 50%, it is important to explain to him that a recent analysis of the Sudden Cardiac Death in Heart Failure Trial showed that patients with an implanted ICD who had an improvement in EF to greater than 35% accrued a similar relative reduction in mortality with ICD therapy as those whose EF remained at 35% or less.[14] There is a scarcity of data in this territory, but the patient needs to understand the potential risks associated with reimplantation or avoiding reimplantation and make a decision accordingly.

In another example, a 45-year-old woman received a dual-chamber pacemaker for persistent tachycardia-bradycardia syndrome after mitral valve repair and maze surgery. Two years later, she develops a device pocket infection with device erosion. Device interrogation reveals a normal sinus rhythm with narrow QRS and no pacing requirements for at least a year. Moreover, she is not on any antiarrhythmic therapies and has not had recurrent episodes of persistent atrial fibrillation. Her heart rate increases appropriately with exercise. Given that her pacing indication has resolved, it is recommended that she undergoes full device extraction without reimplantation.

It is important to also consider the potential emotional impact of removing either pacemaker or ICD therapy. Patients and families sometimes become as emotionally dependent on the device as clinically dependent. If there is time, programming the pacemaker therapy off (not just slower) to assess clinical and emotional dependence and disabling tachycardia detection is wise. There is a potential that a loss of CRT, even if temporary during infection therapy, could cause hemodynamic compromise in some patients. Time needs to be spent with patients and families to address this issue before the extraction procedure.

Considerations for reimplantation after infected cardiovascular implantable electronic device extraction

Timing of cardiovascular implantable electronic device reimplantation If reimplantation is indicated, choosing the right time to reimplant a new device is a crucial component of achieving successful outcomes. The default is to wait as long as possible until the antibiotic course is completed before reimplantation. Ideally, patients should be fully treated and be without any signs of local or systemic infection. Although waiting is easy to accomplish in certain patient groups, such as those with primary prevention ICD without events or sinus node dysfunction, others are device dependent and device support is essential clinically. Examples include pacemaker-dependent patients, CRT responders, and those with secondary prevention ICDs at high risk of ventricular tachyarrhythmias. It is important that the cardiology and infectious disease teams discuss the details of each case in order to achieve the best and safest outcomes for every individual patient. This discussion should include identifying the microorganism involved through blood and device cultures, choosing the right antibiotics, repeating blood cultures, considering the need for transesophageal echocardiography if endocarditis is suspected, evaluating the patients clinically after extraction for signs of local or systemic infection, and finally determining the optimal time for reimplantation (**Fig. 1**).

Pacing-therapy–dependent patients In such patients, reimplantation is preferable after at least 3

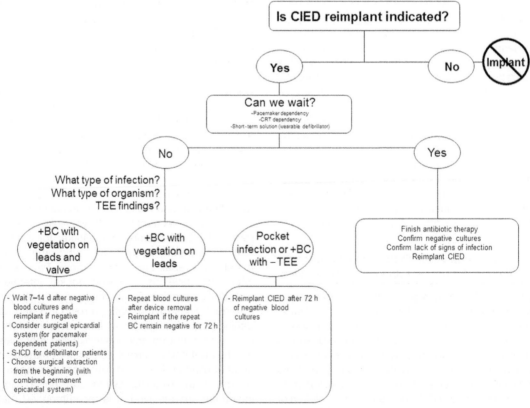

Fig. 1. The decision-making process for CIED reimplantation after lead removal for CIED infection. BC, blood cultures; S-ICD, subcutaneous ICDs; TEE, transesophageal echocardiogram.

to 5 days of negative blood cultures and absence of signs of systemic or local infection.[1] The authors always strive to find an optimal balance between allowing enough time for the infection to clear on one hand and the cost and time associated with prolonging hospitalization along with the risk of infection associated with a temporary transvenous pacemaker lead on the other hand. For example, in patients with complete heart block who undergo extraction for pacemaker infection, a temporary pacemaker is implanted until the patients' blood cultures are negative for 72 hours or more, subsequently clearing them for reimplantation. We must also continue to evaluate the patients daily for the need of immediate reimplantation. In CRT responders, extraction can lead to rapid deterioration of their congestive heart failure (CHF). Although we may initially assume that it is safe for these patients to undergo reimplantation after completing the full antibiotic course for 2 to 4 weeks, some may develop decompensated CHF requiring prompt reimplantation of CRT. This scenario sometimes holds true even for patients who were deemed nonresponders by echo criteria; but once they lose the biventricular pacing, they can deteriorate clinically.

Patients not pacing-therapy dependent Some patients with CIED infection do not depend on their device, such as those with chronotropic incompetence as discussed earlier. The optimal management plan for these patients is to wait until the infection is completely resolved and fully treated with antibiotics. Typically, such patients would be discharged from the hospital to complete their course of antibiotics with close monitoring of their need for a device. After completing the appropriate 2- to 6-week course of antibiotics,[1] depending on the clinical scenario, they return for an outpatient visit. At that time, we should carefully evaluate patients for any signs of persistent infection, such as endocarditis; confirm that they have completed their course of antibiotics; and most importantly discuss with patients the indications for reimplantation allowing them to make a well-informed decision. This time is also a good opportunity to carefully plan the reimplantation procedure and choose what kind of device to reimplant if any.

Temporary bridging to permanent reimplantation after infected cardiovascular implantable electronic device extraction Determining the patients' need for a bridging device to reimplantation is another crucial aspect of the decision-making process in patients undergoing CIED extraction. As the authors discuss earlier, many patients undergoing extraction are not pacing therapy

dependent or do not require reimplantation at all. However, in CIED therapy–dependent patients, a bridge to permanent reimplantation is necessary. In those dependent on pacemakers, an active fixation pacing lead, usually introduced through the internal jugular vein and connected to an external pacing device, is placed before the extraction procedure and can remain in place until reimplantation of a new system. The external device can be taped to the chest wall allowing patient mobility and cardiac-unit rather than coronary-care-unit monitoring.[15] However, in ICD patients without pacing needs who undergo extraction, the decision to bridge requires more careful scrutiny. The recent advent of wearable cardioverter-defibrillators (WCDs) provides a valuable solution in some high-risk patients allowing for simultaneous completion of the antibiotic course and protection from sudden arrhythmic death. A recent study of 21 patients who underwent ICD or CRT-D removal because of infection and were prescribed a WCD showed that one patient had a symptomatic episode of sustained ventricular tachycardia requiring a shock.[16] There are no large studies yet to support using WCD as a bridge in patients with a high-risk of ventricular arrhythmias who underwent extraction; however, it should be considered as a feasible option. Remember there is both the clinical need and also the need to emotionally support patients through this transition. Often the WCD is helpful with this transition.

Type of permanent device to reimplant The final aspect of the decision-making process for CIED reimplantation is deciding what type of permanent device to reimplant. Recent advances in pacing and defibrillation technology have produced new devices, such as leadless pacemakers and subcutaneous ICDs (S-ICD). Two leadless pacemaker systems have been studied, the Nanostim Leadless Pacemaker (Abbott, Lake Bluff, IL, USA) and the Micra Transcatheter Pacing System (Medtronic plc, Minneapolis, MN, USA); they provide a new alternative for single-chamber right ventricular pacing that does not require intravascular leads or pockets.[2,17] The Micra leadless pacemaker (Medtronic plc) is the only one currently approved by the Food and Drug Administration. Despite the current scarcity of evidence, patients with VVI pacing indications who have had a CIED infection and extraction can be considered for the option of leadless pacemaker reimplantation. Leadless pacemakers do not require a pocket, and pocket infections account for close to 60% of all CIED infections.[6] Likewise, patients with ICD infection who require ICD extraction and reimplantation could be considered for an S-ICD, as long as they have no pacing indications. With the lack of endovascular components, S-ICDs avoid the risk of endovascular infections. The rate of infections associated with S-ICD implantation in general is at least similar to transvenous ICD. However, it is important to note that in a study by Boersma and colleagues,[18] all infections related to S-ICDs were local infections and none were systemic. However, there have been no comparative studies between S-ICDs and transvenous ICDs that would allow us to conclude S-ICDs have a clear advantage in terms of minimizing infection risk.

It is also important to consider simplifying patients' devices (ICD to pacemaker) if there is emergence of new clinical conditions, lack of indication for ICD, or patient preference that would obviate a defibrillator and there is still a pacing indication. Patients who are pacemaker dependent and CRT responders who developed a CRT-D infection requiring extraction, but now with advanced age, may prefer not to have a defibrillator. Such patients could be reimplanted with a CRT-P device. Extracting dual-coil ICD leads is associated with higher all-cause mortality within 30 days of extraction; thus, one must make the effort not to reimplant an ICD.[19]

One other consideration is planning reimplantation in patients with CRT. Replacing a coronary sinus (CS) lead in nonresponders is controversial and should be avoided if the potential harm outweighs the benefit. One should be careful about the group of patients who might seem to be nonresponders by echo criteria but can deteriorate quickly after removal of their CRT device. Reimplantation in responders is necessary, and the operator should plan for it meticulously with the goal of reimplanting a new CS in the same branch of the CS as the old one. Reimplantation can be difficult because of thrombosis, injury, or occlusion of the CS and its branches during the extraction procedure. Retaining access to the CS with a guidewire delivered through the extraction sheath lumen can be used to retain access in noninfectious cases when reimplantation is performed during the same procedure.[1] In infectious cases, one may consider performing a CS venogram after extraction in order to better plan for the reimplantation procedure. If reimplantation of a CS lead is technically not feasible, implantation of an epicardial left ventricular lead or His bundle pacing can be considered.

Common practice in pacemaker-dependent patients involves full system extraction followed by placing a temporary pacemaker as a bridge to permanent reimplantation. However, this approach could be challenging, especially among patients who present with endocarditis with bacteremia and vegetations on their leads or tricuspid valves. Some experts have suggested using a single combined procedure of transvenous CIED system extraction and epicardial pacemaker implantation to prevent a prolonged hospital stay associated with bridging. In one study, 160 patients underwent randomization to extraction with an externalized pacemaker and delayed implantation on the contralateral side versus surgical implantation of 2 epicardial ventricular leads with extraction of the infected pacemaker during the same procedure.[20] Both strategies had an excellent success rate and low risk of complications, and the combined procedure approach was associated with a shorter duration of hospital stay. These findings were replicated in another study.[21] Although this approach may be feasible in many patients, the cardiac team has to consider the whole picture and inform patients about the harms versus benefits associated with each strategy. High-volume centers with cardiothoracic surgeons with specific expertise in placement of epicardial pacing leads are integral to achieving good outcomes using this strategy. Additionally, surgical extraction of CIEDs could also be challenging, especially in cases with heavy fibrosis along the SVC. Although the surgical exposure is excellent to remove the intracardiac components and the pocket components, it could be limited for the venous structure from the subclavian vein to the SVC. Leaving a remnant of the lead in the SVC could be detrimental and should be avoided. Therefore, some of these surgical extraction procedures can be performed in a hybrid room with a combination of surgical and transvenous lead extraction techniques.

TECHNICAL CONSIDERATIONS

After discussing all the factors at play during the decision-making process for reimplantation after CIED extraction, several procedural technical details need to be taken into account.

Location of Reimplantation

In CIED extraction for noninfectious indications, a new CIED is usually reimplanted on the same side. This technique usually involves maintaining vascular access after the extraction in order to place the new lead, as discussed earlier. The operator must be cognizant of the fact that extraction can lead to significant injury to the venous walls, particularly in leads greater than 5 years old, as the authors previously discussed.[12] Therefore, the operator should be extra careful with manipulating and advancing the new lead in order to avoid vascular wall perforation. A long peel-away sheath, usually 20 to 24 cm, is usually used to introduce the lead beyond the SVC junction to the right atrium. In patients who undergo extraction for an infectious indication, venous access should be performed in an alternative location, such as the contralateral side (internal jugular, subclavian, axillary or cephalic), the iliac vein, transatrial approach, or using epicardial or subcutaneous implantation, as the authors have previously discussed.[1] In cases of valve endocarditis accompanying CIED infection, epicardial permanent pacemaker system could be implanted for patients who need pacing and consideration of an S-ICD for patients who need ICD without a pacing indication in order to decrease the chances of recurrent endocarditis. A transesophageal echocardiogram (TEE) is advisable both before and after transvenous lead extraction to assess the preoperative presence of vegetations and the potential for ghosts, which are the fibrotic remnants produced by shearing the scar tissue off of the lead body but left behind. Whether the TEE findings are interpreted as vegetations will impact both the timing and approach to device reimplantation.

Minimal Infection Risk Practices

CIED infection is associated with high morbidity and mortality. Thus, we must maintain a high level of sterility and use best-practice measures to avoid procedure-related reinfection during reimplantation. This endeavor can be daunting when reimplanting devices immediately after extraction given the length of the procedure and the need to use multiple extraction and reimplantation tools. The operator must ensure sterile conditions of the surgical field, use of optimal antiseptic preparation of the skin across a wide area covering the whole surgical site, and use of systemic antibiotic therapy administered before the surgical incision. Some observational studies have shown that perioperative antibiotic administration 1 hour before the procedure significantly reduced the incidence of device infection.[22,23] A randomized clinical trial comparing prophylactic antibiotics with placebo showed significant reduction in device infection in the antibiotic arm, thus, making it standard practice.[24] A first-generation cephalosporin or vancomycin is commonly used. There is no evidence to support any additional antibiotic therapy; however, the Prevention of Arrhythmia Device Infection Trial (PADIT) is evaluating 2 strategies, one using conventional prophylactic antibiotic at the time of the CIED procedure and a second that involves preprocedure and postprocedure antibiotic therapy.[25] It is important to note that some measures, such as povidone iodine ointment, neomycin ointment, and antiseptic pads, have shown no significant added benefit in preventing CIED infection.[26] Although a nonabsorbable antibacterial envelope placed around the device generator has shown significant reduction in CIED infection in a nonrandomized study,[27] these envelopes have been associated with significant pocket fibrosis and adhesions that may make future generator changes difficult. The new generation of the antibacterial envelope is fully absorbable and seems to be associated with a lower incidence of CIED-related pocket infections in high-risk patients.[28] A large multicenter international randomized trial is currently in progress assessing the efficacy of the absorbable antibiotic envelope in reducing CIED infection among patients undergoing device replacement or upgrades.[29]

SUMMARY

The increasing number of CIEDs implanted in younger patients is leading to an increase in the number of CIEDs worldwide and consequently an increasing rate of CIED complications and infection. Therefore, we have witnessed an upsurge in CIED extraction procedures in the last few years. Reimplantation after extraction is a multifaceted decision process that should involve the collaboration of a multidisciplinary team including cardiac electrophysiology, cardiology, cardiac surgery, and infectious disease. In each individual case, the multidisciplinary team must discuss the patients' indication for reimplantation, optimal timing for reimplantation, whether a bridging device is indicated, and finally what type of new permanent device to reimplant and where. The plan must be discussed with patients, and their wishes must be taken into consideration before the extraction procedure. Meticulous preprocedural decision-making coupled with careful technical planning ensure favorable and safe long-term outcomes for these patients.

REFERENCES

1. Kusumoto FM, Schoenfeld MH, Wilkoff BL, et al. 2017 HRS expert consensus statement on cardiovascular implantable electronic device lead management and extraction. Heart Rhythm 2017; 14(12):e503–51.
2. Tarakji KG, Ellis CR, Defaye P, et al. Cardiac implantable electronic device infection in patients at risk. Arrhythm Electrophysiol Rev 2016;5(1):65–71.
3. Voigt A, Shalaby A, Saba S. Continued rise in rates of cardiovascular implantable electronic device infections in the United States: temporal trends and causative insights. Pacing Clin Electrophysiol 2010;33(4):414–9.

4. Greenspon AJ, Patel JD, Lau E, et al. 16-year trends in the infection burden for pacemakers and implantable cardioverter-defibrillators in the United States 1993 to 2008. J Am Coll Cardiol 2011;58(10):1001–6.

5. Eckstein J, Koller MT, Zabel M, et al. Necessity for surgical revision of defibrillator leads implanted long-term: causes and management. Circulation 2008;117(21):2727–33.

6. Tarakji KG, Chan EJ, Cantillon DJ, et al. Cardiac implantable electronic device infections: presentation, management, and patient outcomes. Heart Rhythm 2010;7(8):1043–7.

7. Sohail MR, Uslan DZ, Khan AH, et al. Management and outcome of permanent pacemaker and implantable cardioverter-defibrillator infections. J Am Coll Cardiol 2007;49(18):1851–9.

8. Al-Hijji MA, Killu AM, Yousefian O, et al. Outcomes of lead extraction without subsequent device reimplantation. Europace 2017;19(9):1527–34.

9. Pokorney SD, Mi X, Lewis RK, et al. Outcomes associated with extraction versus capping and abandoning pacing and defibrillator leads. Circulation 2017; 136(15):1387–95.

10. Barakat AF, Wazni OM, Tarakji K, et al. Transvenous lead extraction at the time of cardiac implantable electronic device upgrade: complexity, safety, and outcomes. Heart Rhythm 2017;14(12):1807–11.

11. Hussein AA, Tarakji KG, Martin DO, et al. Cardiac implantable electronic device infections: added complexity and suboptimal outcomes with previously abandoned leads. JACC Clin Electrophysiol 2017;3(1):1–9.

12. Tarakji KG, Saliba W, Markabawi D, et al. Unrecognized venous injuries after cardiac implantable electronic device transvenous lead extraction. Heart Rhythm 2017. https://doi.org/10.1016/j.hrthm.2017.11.008.

13. Tarakji KG, Wazni OM, Harb S, et al. Risk factors for 1-year mortality among patients with cardiac implantable electronic device infection undergoing transvenous lead extraction: the impact of the infection type and the presence of vegetation on survival. Europace 2014;16(10):1490–5.

14. Adabag S, Patton KK, Buxton AE, et al. Association of implantable cardioverter defibrillators with survival in patients with and without improved ejection fraction. JAMA Cardiol 2017;2(7):767–74.

15. Braun MU, Rauwolf T, Bock M, et al. Percutaneous lead implantation connected to an external device in stimulation-dependent patients with systemic infection–a prospective and controlled study. Pacing Clin Electrophysiol 2006;29(8):875–9.

16. Castro L, Pecha S, Linder M, et al. The wearable cardioverter defibrillator as a bridge to reimplantation in patients with ICD or CRT-D-related infections. J Cardiothorac Surg 2017;12(1):99.

17. Gold MR. Are leadless pacemakers a niche or the future of device therapy? J Am Coll Cardiol 2015; 65(15):1505–8.

18. Boersma L, Burke MC, Neuzil P, et al. Infection and mortality after implantation of a subcutaneous ICD after transvenous ICD extraction. Heart Rhythm 2016;13(1):157–64.

19. Brunner MP, Cronin EM, Duarte VE, et al. Clinical predictors of adverse patient outcomes in an experience of more than 5000 chronic endovascular pacemaker and defibrillator lead extractions. Heart Rhythm 2014;11(5):799–805.

20. Amraoui S, Sohal M, Li A, et al. Comparison of delayed transvenous reimplantation and immediate surgical epicardial approach in pacing-dependent patients undergoing extraction of infected permanent pacemakers. Heart Rhythm 2015;12(6):1209–15.

21. Perrin T, Maille B, Lemoine C, et al. Comparison of epicardial vs. endocardial reimplantation in pacemaker-dependent patients with device infection. Europace 2017. https://doi.org/10.1093/europace/eux111.

22. Polyzos KA, Konstantelias AA, Falagas ME. Risk factors for cardiac implantable electronic device infection: a systematic review and meta-analysis. Europace 2015;17(5):767–77.

23. Darouiche R, Mosier M, Voigt J. Antibiotics and antiseptics to prevent infection in cardiac rhythm management device implantation surgery. Pacing Clin Electrophysiol 2012;35(11):1348–60.

24. de Oliveira JC, Martinelli M, Nishioka SAD, et al. Efficacy of antibiotic prophylaxis before the implantation of pacemakers and cardioverter-defibrillators: results of a large, prospective, randomized, double-blinded, placebo-controlled trial. Circ Arrhythm Electrophysiol 2009;2(1):29–34.

25. Connolly SJ, Philippon F, Longtin Y, et al. Randomized cluster crossover trials for reliable, efficient, comparative effectiveness testing: design of the Prevention of Arrhythmia Device Infection Trial (PADIT). Can J Cardiol 2013;29(6):652–8.

26. Khalighi K, Aung TT, Elmi F. The role of prophylaxis topical antibiotics in cardiac device implantation. Pacing Clin Electrophysiol 2014;37(3):304–11.

27. Mittal S, Shaw RE, Michel K, et al. Cardiac implantable electronic device infections: incidence, risk factors, and the effect of the AigisRx antibacterial envelope. Heart Rhythm 2014;11(4):595–601.

28. Kolek MJ, Patel NJ, Clair WK, et al. Efficacy of a bio-absorbable antibacterial envelope to prevent cardiac implantable electronic device infections in high-risk subjects. J Cardiovasc Electrophysiol 2015;26(10):1111–6.

29. Tarakji KG, Mittal S, Kennergren C, et al. Worldwide randomized antibiotic envelope infection prevention trial (WRAP-IT). Am Heart J 2016;180:12–21.

Venoplasty and Stenting

Kevin P. Jackson, MD

KEYWORDS

- Lead management • Occlusion • Angioplasty • Cardiac resynchronization therapy

KEY POINTS

- Partial or complete venous obstruction at the time of lead revision or device upgrade is frequently encountered. Successful strategies to overcome this problem can significantly impact patient outcomes.
- Subclavian venoplasty can be performed safely and effectively by the implanting physician with a basic understanding of the tools and techniques required.
- Coronary sinus venoplasty can be performed when a stenotic vessel significantly impedes lead placement in the desired target branch. Stenting for lead stabilization is rarely required in the era of modern lead design and fixation.

 Video content accompanies this article at http://www.cardiacep.theclinics.com/.

INTRODUCTION

With expanding indications for cardiac resynchronization therapy (CRT) and increased survival of patients with cardiovascular disease, the need for lead revision or lead addition in the setting of existing cardiovascular implantable electronic devices (CIEDs) is likely to increase.[1] Venous access in the situation of partial or complete vessel occlusion can be a significant barrier to a successful procedural outcome. Percutaneous options, including subclavian venoplasty, can reduce the need for significantly more invasive and morbid procedures. However, this procedure is rarely performed by electrophysiologists, as the skillset required is generally not taught during formal training.

WHAT IS THE INCIDENCE OF VENOUS OBSTRUCTION?

Although primary venous obstruction at the time of de novo device implantation is rare, the incidence of partial or complete obstruction from preexisting leads or prior instrumentation is fairly common. In approximately 25% of patients with an existing CIED, there is venous obstruction to some degree, with severe or complete obstruction estimated in 10% of patients. Vessel stenosis usually occurs peripherally in the subclavian vein; however, central obstruction or obstruction at multiple locations is not uncommon. Factors associated with a higher chance of stenosis include greater total lead diameter, time since implant, and the presence of multiple leads.[2] Given the frequency of venous obstruction, a preprocedure peripheral venogram or noninvasive ultrasound should be considered in all patients undergoing a system upgrade or lead revision. Local venography from the access needle or a small catheter placed in the axillary vein may reveal a patent tract not apparent on peripheral venography and can help guidewire manipulation across the occlusion (**Fig. 1**).

WHAT ARE THE OPTIONS WHEN VENOUS OBSTRUCTION IS FOUND?

Historically, cardiac device implantation was performed by surgeons; therefore, venous obstruction was generally managed with surgical techniques, including tunneling or epicardial lead

Disclosure Statement: Research grants, consulting, and advisory board from Medtronic (K.P. Jackson).
Department of Medicine, Division of Cardiology, Duke University Medical Center, Box 3816, Durham, NC 27710, USA
E-mail address: k.j@duke.edu

Card Electrophysiol Clin 10 (2018) 675–680
https://doi.org/10.1016/j.ccep.2018.07.005

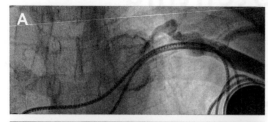
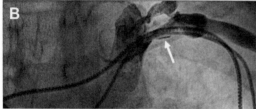

Fig. 1. Local contrast injection can help identify a patent tract through a partially occluded subclavian vessel. In panel (*A*) contrast injected through a peripheral IV in the left arm suggests complete occlusion of the vein with formation of collateral drainage. In panel (*B*) local injection through the access needle in the axillary vein demonstrates a patent tract (*arrow*), which can help guidewire manipulation across the occlusion.

placement. As the procedure moved to the purview of interventional cardiology and electrophysiology, management options for venous obstruction have evolved (**Box 1**).

Of these options, abandonment of an existing, functioning system with new implantation on the contralateral side is often the least desirable, because of the placement of redundant leads and the risk of future bilateral venous obstruction. Tunneling of a new CIED lead across the sternum from the contralateral side, such as a left ventricular (LV) lead during CRT upgrade, is feasible even in patients with prior sternotomy, however, similarly may compromise future venous access procedures. Surgical (epicardial) placement of LV

leads results in increased morbidity and prolonged hospital stay compared with transvenous lead placement. In a series of 452 patients undergoing CRT implantation, 10% failed transvenous LV lead insertion and underwent epicardial lead placement. Acute renal injury and infection were significantly higher in this group compared with matched controls (26.2% vs 4.9%: $P = .0004$; 11.9% vs 2.4%: $P = .03$, respectively).[3] The REPLACE study examined outcomes in patients undergoing CIED replacement including 407 patients with a planned upgrade to CRT.[4] In this registry, there were 4 deaths from among the 48 patients (8% mortality) who went for an epicardial lead following a failed transvenous approach.

The choice between lead extraction with retained access versus subclavian venoplasty with preservation of the existing system often depends on operator expertise and familiarity with the procedure.[5] In the case of replacement of a redundant lead (eg, new defibrillator lead in the setting of a lead fracture), especially in a younger patient, extraction of unused hardware may be preferable. In the situation of a system upgrade (eg, addition of an LV lead for CRT upgrade), venoplasty avoids the necessity of sacrificing an otherwise functioning lead. The skill set required to perform successful venoplasty involves basic interventional knowledge and technical skills, which are not typically acquired during formal cardiac electrophysiology training; therefore, it may be advisable to include a physician with formal training in interventional cardiology or interventional radiology with the introduction of this procedure.

THE BASICS OF SUBCLAVIAN VENOPLASTY

When an occluded subclavian vein is encountered and venoplasty is planned, a standard tool set should be made available (**Box 2**). The first step is obtaining vessel access to allow adequate wire and catheter manipulation. For many peripheral occlusions, these tasks are easier if the axillary vein is accessed over the second thoracic rib, although final implantation of a lead with this more lateral access may increase the risk of chronic flexing injury. After successful vein puncture with the needle, a standard 0.035-in J-wire is inserted up to the point of occlusion and the needle is removed. Next, a small 5-F sheath is inserted over the wire to maintain access. A Y-adaptor can be attached to the end of the sheath, thereby allowing simultaneous wire manipulation and contrast injection. Once the sheath is in place, a short (150–180 cm) 0.035-in angled glide wire is introduced and the vessel is

---

Box 1
Management options for venous occlusion encountered during device implant, lead revision, or system upgrade

- Abandon access and implant system on contralateral side
- Tunnel new lead (eg, left ventricular lead) across the sternum from contralateral side
- Epicardial (surgical) lead implant
- Mechanical or laser lead extraction of redundant lead with retained access
- Subclavian venoplasty

> **Box 2**
> **Key elements and tools for subclavian venoplasty**
>
> - Obtain access lateral to the occlusion and inject contrast locally to find a potential tract across the lesion.
> - Use a 0.035-in angled glide wire and wire torque device to cross the lesion.
> - A 4-F hydrophilic support catheter can provide wire support across long occlusions and allows a platform to exchange for an extra-stiff wire once the lesion is crossed.
> - Confirm the wire is intraluminal (advanced to IVC or pulmonary artery) before inserting the balloon.
> - Use a 6 mm × 40-mm noncompliant peripheral angioplasty balloon for a single lead implant or up to a 9-mm balloon when multiple leads are required.
> - Inflate the balloon to rated burst pressure or until the waist is eliminated.

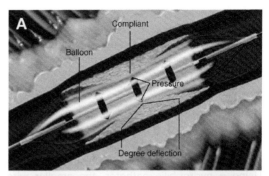

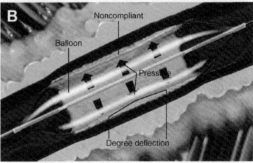

Fig. 2. Comparison of the deformation profile between a compliant (*A*) and noncompliant (*B*) balloon. (*From* Jackson KP, Lewis RL. Interventional techniques for device implantation. In: Ellenbogen KA, Wilkoff BL, editors. Clinical cardiac pacing, defibrillation and resynchronization therapy. 5th edition. Philadelphia (PA): Elsevier; 2015. p. 846; with permission.)

probed for a tract through the occlusion. A wire torque device is helpful in allowing fine manipulation of the wire tip. In long occlusions, use of a hydrophilic sheath (support catheter) allows advancement over the wire as progress is made through the occlusion. Once the lesion is crossed, the operator must confirm that the wire or catheter has reentered the true lumen of the vein before proceeding with balloon venoplasty. This confirmation is done by advancing the wire into the inferior vena cava (IVC) or the pulmonary artery or by injecting a small amount of contrast through the support catheter.

Before starting venoplasty, it is advisable to exchange the 0.035-in hydrophilic glide wire for a 0.035-in extrastiff wire using the hydrophilic support catheter. This exchange allows a more stable platform for balloon and sheath advancement. Balloon dilation of an occluded subclavian vein is most readily accomplished with the use of a noncompliant, 6- to 9-mm-diameter peripheral angioplasty balloon. Whereas a compliant balloon may stretch on either side of a lesion, a noncompliant balloon concentrates the force more uniformly (**Fig. 2**). With difficult lesions, an ultranoncompliant (Kevlar), high-pressure balloon may be used. The peripheral angioplasty balloon is advanced over the wire to the most central occlusion and inflated to the nominal pressure (listed on the package). At the nominal pressure, the balloon reaches the labeled diameter. If the waist does not open, inflation pressure is increased until rated burst pressure is reached (**Fig. 3**). Serial, overlapping

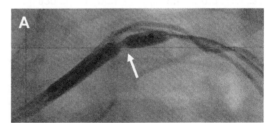

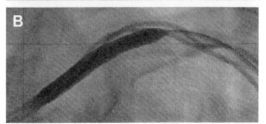

Fig. 3. Example of subclavian venoplasty. In panel (*A*), a 7-mm-diameter by 40-mm-length noncompliant balloon (Ultraverse, Bard Peripheral Vascular, Tempe, AZ) is advanced across the stenosis and inflated. Note the waist evident on initial inflation (*arrow*). In panel (*B*), at nominal pressure, the waist is completely eliminated. (*Courtesy of* Bard Peripheral Vascular, Inc, Tempe, AZ.)

inflations are performed over the length of the occlusion (Video 1). Once the occluded vessel is successfully opened, vessel stenting is not required and should be avoided because of the entrapment of the existing leads.

On occasion, a narrow or total occlusion cannot be crossed by a 0.035-in wire or peripheral angioplasty balloon. In this situation, a smaller 0.014-in or 0.018-in hydrophilic wire can be used and a coronary balloon (typically 2- to 3-mm diameter) is used to predilate the lesion. Using a hydrophilic catheter, the smaller wire can then be exchanged for a 0.035-in extrastiff wire allowing advancement and inflation of the larger peripheral angioplasty balloon. Successful advancement of a coronary sinus (CS) sheath for LV lead delivery typically requires dilation with a 6-mm-diameter balloon. When implantation of multiple new leads is required, a balloon diameter up to 9 mm may be required. Finally, if the stenosis cannot be crossed with any caliber wire, special tools that allow microdissection or radiofrequency perforation of the occlusion can be used.[6]

COMPLICATIONS OF SUBCLAVIAN VENOPLASTY

Balloon dilation of a subclavian stenosis can be safely performed once the wire crossing the lesion is confirmed to be intraluminal as described earlier. Failure to do so could result in vessel rupture with rapid hemodynamic collapse. Thankfully, this seems to be quite rare. In a large published series on 373 patients undergoing subclavian venoplasty, Worley and colleagues[7] reported no significant clinical complications associated with the procedure. Importantly, no existing leads were reported damaged. Contrast staining related to attempts to manipulate a wire through a stenosis is common and generally inconsequential. Even in the rare situation of balloon rupture, contrast extravasation into surrounding fibrotic tissue is seen; but hemodynamic sequelae have not been reported.

CONTRAST USE IN HIGH-RISK PATIENTS

Visualization of the obstruction with contrast, both initially and during wire and catheter advancement, is essential to successful subclavian venoplasty. In the case of a CRT upgrade with the addition of an LV lead, the operator must consider that contrast may be used at multiple steps of the procedure, including the peripheral and local subclavian venogram, CS access and venogram, as well as target branch access.

Renal insufficiency is present at baseline in more than half of patients with heart failure. Although uncommon in most situations, contrast-induced nephropathy (CIN) can be a significant complication of the CRT procedure and is associated with increased morbidity and mortality and extended hospital stay.[8] After exposure to contrast, the kidneys concentrate contrast material in the urinary space within the renal tubules, releasing nitric oxide from endothelial cells and triggering a transient vasodilation. This result is followed by prolonged vasoconstriction lasting hours or days, which may cause tubular cell damage. The cornerstone of CIN prevention is adequate hydration, which increases the urine flow rate and limits the time of contact between the contrast media and the tubular epithelial cells. Intravenous isotonic sodium chloride (0.9%) is used preferentially, as randomized trial data have shown no additional benefit with the infusion of sodium bicarbonate or pretreatment with oral acetylcysteine.[9]

Even in patients with heart failure, renal insufficiency, diabetes, or other high-risk features, intravenous contrast can be used safely if several key points are considered:

- It is more important to focus on mitigating the risk of contrast rather than minimizing or eliminating its use.
- Bolus hydration with isotonic fluid (normal saline) at an infusion rate of 3 mL/kg starting 1 hour before the procedure followed by 1 mL/kg during and 6 hours after the procedure is highly effective at preventing CIN.
- Fluid overload from intravenous hydration in patients with heart failure is generally easier to manage than acute renal failure.

VENOPLASTY VERSUS PROGRESSIVE DILATORS

Operators unfamiliar with the tools and techniques of subclavian venoplasty may opt to serially dilate a subclavian stenosis with progressively larger dilators. There are several disadvantages and potential perils with this approach. Firstly, although only a peripheral occlusion may be apparent at the time of venography, nearly a quarter of patients will have an additional, more central occlusion that needs to be addressed. Even in the presence of a solitary stenosis, progressive dilation rarely relieves the obstruction enough to allow the unrestricted catheter movement required for successful CS cannulation and LV lead placement. Finally, when multiple new leads are required, failure to adequately open a stenosis may result in additional difficulty manipulating catheters and leads, which can be particularly time consuming.

CORONARY SINUS VENOPLASTY AND STENTING FOR LEFT VENTRICULAR LEAD PLACEMENT

Rarely, the implanting physician encounters a stenotic lesion in the main body of the CS or the target vein, preventing placement of the LV lead in the optimal location. Percutaneous coronary venoplasty of the main CS, stenotic target veins, or collateral vessels between 2 veins can be performed, reducing the need to accept a suboptimal LV lead position or implant failure. In a retrospective series of 705 patients undergoing CRT implantation, 3.5% required venoplasty of the CS ostium, main CS, or target branch for successful lead placement. For target branch venoplasty, a small-caliber (0.014 in) hydrophilic wire is advanced through the stenosis and a compliant (8–12 atmospheric rated burst pressure) coronary angioplasty balloon is selected. The choice of balloon size is based on the estimated vessel diameter as well as the lead profile and is typically between 2 and 3 mm. As with the reported experience for subclavian venoplasty, complications seem to be rare. However, venous dissection or vessel rupture can occur with resultant hemopericardium and tamponade. In patients with prior cardiac surgery, pericardial adhesions may limit any significant bleeding from the low-pressure venous system. In patients without prior cardiac surgery, a careful risk-to-benefit assessment should be performed before CS venoplasty.

Stent placement in the branch vessels of the CS can be performed in the situation of residual stenosis after balloon inflation preventing lead advancement or as a method to stabilize the lead position. In a large single-center experience on CS stenting, the procedure was successful in 312 out of 317 patients (97%) with rare reported complications.[10] Eventual lead extraction was required in 3 patients because of device infection with no reported difficulty in removal with simple traction. Although certainly feasible, with the advent of widely spaced quadripolar LV leads that allow the tip to be wedged in smaller vessels as well as newer active fixation leads, stenting for lead stabilization is unlikely to be required.[11]

SUMMARY

Venous obstruction encountered during lead revision or device upgrade in patients with existing CIEDs requires careful consideration.

Subclavian venoplasty allows preservation of functioning hardware and can be performed safely by the implanting physician with a basic understanding of the tools and techniques required.

SUPPLEMENTARY DATA

Supplementary data related to this article can be found online at https://doi.org/10.1016/j.ccep.2018.07.005.

REFERENCES

1. Epstein AE, DiMarco JP, Ellenbogen KA, et al. 2012 ACCF/AHA/HRS focused update incorporated into the ACCF/AHA/HRS 2008 guidelines for device-based therapy of cardiac rhythm abnormalities: a report of the American College of Cardiology Foundation/American Heart Association Task Force on Practice Guidelines and the Heart Rhythm Society. J Am Coll Cardiol 2013;61(3): e6–75.
2. Abu-El-Haija B, Bhave PD, Campbell DN, et al. Venous Stenosis after transvenous lead placement: a study of outcomes and risk factors in 212 consecutive patients. J Am Heart Assoc 2015;4(8): e001878.
3. Ailawadi G, Lapar DJ, Swenson BR, et al. Surgically placed left ventricular leads provide similar outcomes to percutaneous leads in patients with failed coronary sinus lead placement. Heart Rhythm 2010; 7(5):619–25.
4. Poole JE, Gleva MJ, Mela T, et al. Complication rates associated with pacemaker or implantable cardioverter-defibrillator generator replacements and upgrade procedures: results from the REPLACE registry. Circulation 2010;122(16): 1553–61.
5. Kusumoto FM, Schoenfeld MH, Wilkoff BL, et al. 2017 HRS expert consensus statement on cardiovascular implantable electronic device lead management and extraction. Heart Rhythm 2017; 14(12):e503–51.
6. Baerlocher MO, Asch MR, Myers A. Successful recanalization of a longstanding complete left subclavian vein occlusion by radiofrequency perforation with use of a radiofrequency guide wire. J Vasc Interv Radiol 2006;17(10):1703–6.
7. Worley SJ, Gohn DC, Pulliam RW, et al. Subclavian venoplasty by the implanting physicians in 373 patients over 11 years. Heart Rhythm 2011;8(4): 526–33.
8. Cowburn PJ, Patel H, Pipes RR, et al. Contrast nephropathy post cardiac resynchronization therapy: an under-recognized complication with

important morbidity. Eur J Heart Fail 2005;7(5): 899–903.

9. Weisbord SD, Gallagher M, Jneid H, et al. Outcomes after angiography with sodium bicarbonate and acetylcysteine. N Engl J Med 2018;378(7): 603–14.

10. Geller L, Szilagyi S, Zima E, et al. Long-term experience with coronary sinus side branch stenting to stabilize left ventricular electrode position. Heart Rhythm 2011;8(6):845–50.

11. Keilegavlen H, Hovstad T, Faerestrand S. Active fixation of a thin transvenous left-ventricular lead by a side helix facilitates targeted and stable placement in cardiac resynchronization therapy. Europace 2016;18(8): 1235–40.

Palliation and Nonextraction Approaches

Charles J. Love, MD, FHRS, CCDS

KEYWORDS

- Infected pacemaker • Infected defibrillator • Palliation of CIED infection

KEY POINTS

- A team approach using the electrophysiologist, surgeons, infectious disease consultants, and wound care experts is ideal.
- Obtain fluid, blood, and tissue cultures before starting antibiotic therapy.
- Use targeted antibiotic therapy once the infecting organisms are known.
- Whenever possible, full debridement of all infected tissue and skin edges should be performed.
- Assure excellent hemostasis following wound debridement.
- Consider whether the realistic goal should be palliation or cure and then choose the best treatment options.

Definitive treatment of infections involving cardiac implantable electronic devices (CIED) nearly always requires the removal of all prosthetic material from the implant site and vasculature. This is true unless one is dealing with a superficial skin/wound infection. For infections involving the intravascular portion of the system, leaving behind a small remnant in the heart that is encased in fibrotic material also routinely results in a clinical success. However, there are occasionally situations where lead extraction is not available, not possible, or not in the best interest of the patient.

There are some areas of the world where access to advanced tools, procedural techniques, and experienced medical personnel is not available. For some patients, the leads may be so encased in calcified tissue as to make transvenous extraction, and even open surgical extraction, exceedingly difficult or impossible. Finally, there are some patients for whom system removal does not make sense based on the risk/benefit ratio

given their individual circumstance. For example, this might be a patient in the last year (or less) of life, a patient who is extremely frail with very old leads in place, or one that has multiple morbidities, so as to make the procedure prohibitively dangerous (**Fig. 1**).

The options for patients who cannot or should not have their leads extracted are limited. These are listed in **Box 1**.

These options are not mutually exclusive and should be considered individually or in some combination to achieve the therapeutic goal. Given the complex nature of determining the optimal approach to any individual patient, working with a team of informed heath care professionals is optimal. **Box 2** lists a core group of consultants who may be considered as part of the treatment team. It is worthwhile for this group of experts to develop a close working relationship, so that when such cases arise, all will have an understanding of CIED centric case management.

Disclosure Statement: Consulting fees from Abbott Medical, Convatec, Biotronik, Boston Scientific, Medtronic, Philips Medical.
Johns Hopkins Hospital, 600 North Wolfe Street, Carnegie 592B, Baltimore, MD 21287, USA
E-mail address: cjlovemd@gmail.com

Card Electrophysiol Clin 10 (2018) 681–687
https://doi.org/10.1016/j.ccep.2018.05.002

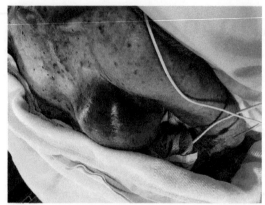

Fig. 1. Picture of an infected pacemaker pocket (*Staphylococcus epidermidis*) in a 101-year-old woman who weighed 87 pounds. Her initial pacemaker was placed in 1986 and she was pacemaker dependent. She developed an infected pacemaker pocket infection without evidence of a systemic infection. After discussion of the options with her and her family, a decision was made to perform a palliative procedure by doing a pocket debridement and relocation, followed by chronic antibiotics to suppress the organism.

CHRONIC SUPPRESSIVE ANTIBIOTIC THERAPY

Long-term treatment of a CIED infection may be useful either alone or in combination with one or more of the other options noted in **Box 1**. Intravascular infections such as lead-associated endocarditis or persistent bacteremia with recurrent sepsis may be managed with chronic antibiotic therapy delivered either orally or intravenously.[1] Although there are rare case reports of success in eradicating intravascular infections with antibiotics alone, this is uncommon. The natural course of events is a recurrence of infection soon after antibiotics are discontinued. However, palliation using continuous, long-term antibiotic therapy may allow for the patient to continue with a reasonable

---

Box 1
Management options when lead extraction cannot or should not be performed

- Chronic suppressive antibiotic therapy
- Pocket debridement with device reimplant at the same site
- Pocket relocation (deeper or adjacent to infected site) with device reimplant
- Chronic open drainage
- Closed pocket irrigation
- Vacuum-assisted wound closure
- Device removal with lead abandonment

Box 2
Potential consultants to be included in infected CIED management

- Cardiac Electrophysiologist
- Cardiac Surgeon
- Infectious Disease Expert
- Plastic Surgeon
- Wound Care Service

---

quality of life. Complications of this approach include evolving resistance of the organisms to the antibiotic therapy, gastrointestinal complications, and *Clostridium difficile* infection. One study showed a 22% complication rate in patients receiving long-term antibiotic therapy.[1]

Unfortunately, initial therapy for device pocket infection using antibiotics alone is almost universally insufficient.[2] This is because of the presence of an abscess and the inability of antibiotics to penetrate and have an effect on the pathologic organisms within the closed space. In most cases, when the pocket is inflamed and contains pus, it must be opened, drained, and debrided as described later in this article. Closure may be possible with continued long-term antibiotic therapy after aggressive wound management has been undertaken.[3]

Initial antibiotic therapy should be broad spectrum and at the very least have coverage for both coagulase-positive and coagulase-negative Staphylococcus organisms (including methicillin resistant strains). It is also prudent to cover Gram-negative organisms. Other pathologic organisms are sufficiently uncommon (eg, mycobacterium, fungus) that it is not reasonable to proactively administer empirical therapy unless there is a high degree of suspicion for an atypical infection. It cannot be overemphasized how important it is to obtain cultures from the infected area and from the bloodstream before initiation of antibiotics. Obtaining cultures from blood and (if possible) from the pocket fluid and tissue before antibiotics are administered will allow for targeted and specific antibiotic therapy to be delivered. Well-meaning clinicians who start antibiotics early, frequently cause culture-negative evaluations to occur complicating therapeutic decision-making regarding antibiotic choice. The result may be the need to use more toxic or broad-spectrum antibiotics to manage the patient, causing the potential for more side effects and the emergence of more drug-resistant bacteria.

In some cases, oral antibiotic therapy may be sufficient for chronic suppression.[4,5] Trimethoprim-sulfamethoxazole is used frequently to help suppress susceptible forms of Staphylococcus. Rifampin may also be useful as an oral agent. Patients on chronic hemodialysis are often treated with intravenous vancomycin delivered during a dialysis session.[6] Ultimately, the choice of antibiotic to be used should be made in consultation with an expert on the infectious disease.

POCKET DEBRIDEMENT

When the device pocket is infected, if not already open, it must be incised and drained to allow exit of purulent material.[3,7] Unfortunately, drainage alone is nearly always insufficient given there is a foreign body present within the abscess. If the wound is already open due to an erosion or wound dehiscence, an incision is made to encompass the infected or thinned skin area. This will allow for primary closure of healthy skin edges at the end of the procedure.

The device must be removed from the pocket and the lead system carefully dissected free from the pocket tissue to the suturing sleeve. Some have recommended that the suturing sleeve and suture material be removed as well, to reduce the potential space where the infecting organisms can avoid exposure to antiseptic and antibiotic agents. If there are any other foreign bodies or elements of the pacing system (eg, older buried leads, lead caps, tie down sutures), these must be dissected free and removed (if possible) or exposed for decontamination.

When possible, the infected tissues should be excised and debrided as completely as possible, thus exposing healthy tissue. This may not be possible on the anterior portion of the pocket when there is little to no subcutaneous tissue between the infected pocket and the skin. This lack of tissue is frequently seen in thin patients, when the device was placed in a very superficial tissue plane, or if the infection is extensive or has caused significant thinning of the subcutaneous tissues. If debridement removes too much of the tissue between the skin and deeper tissues, the blood supply to the skin is compromised and it will eventually slough off. A skin flap may then be necessary to resolve the new problem.

Full debridement will remove much of the dead and infected tissue, thus "debulking" the tissue burden affected by the pathologic process. Attempts at "sterilization" of the leads and device to be left in the pocket along with copious irrigation are described by all accounts of localized pocket debridement. The type of irrigation described varies significantly. Typically, a dilute antiseptic solution such as povidone-iodine is used to irrigate and in many cases to scrub and disinfect the

device and exposed portion of the lead system. Another method uses 3% hydrogen peroxide to help disinfect the pocket and device. An antibiotic solution may be used alone as an alternative, although it is not as effective as the latter options to sterilize the hardware. Various antibiotics are described and include vancomycin, cefazolin, bacitracin, and a combination of bacitracin–polymyxin–neomycin, as well as other agents.[8–12]

The use of pulsed lavage with a specialized irrigation tool such as the Stryker Interpule system (Stryker, Inc, Kalamazoo MI, USA) has been found to be effective in helping to loosen infected and necrotic tissues that remain after surgical debridement is complete (**Fig. 2**). Normal saline, dilute povidone-iodine, or an antibiotic solution is delivered in a high-pressure, pulsed stream with suction to remove the delivered fluid and debris.[6–8,12,13]

Hemostasis is extremely important when debridement is performed. Submuscular and intramuscular pockets in particular can be a challenge due to difficulty visualizing the source of bleeding and the presence of extensive "oozing" from the muscle fibers. The use of hemostatic agents such as topical thrombin, methylcellulose, and human gelatin-thrombin matrix type products in infected areas may not be advisable. Advanced cautery systems such as the Aquamantys (Medtronic, Inc. Minneapolis, USA) that cauterizes a large area may be useful to achieve hemostasis in these challenging anatomic areas (**Fig. 3**).

Once the pocket has been prepared, hemostasis has been assured, and the device and extravascular portion of the lead system is then scrubbed with an antiseptic solution as best as possible, then the system is placed back into the

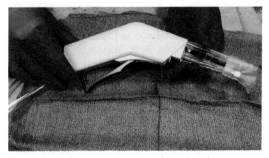

Fig. 2. Pulsed lavage system used to provide a pressurized, pulsed irrigation of infected areas with simultaneous suctioning of the fluid. The system may be used with an antiseptic solution or antibiotic and may provide a more effective method of cleaning out infected areas after surgical debridement. Stryker Interpulse. (*Courtesy of* Stryker Inc, Kalamazoo, MI; with permission.)

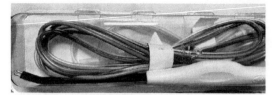

Fig. 3. Aquamantys cautery device (Medtronic, Inc. Minneapolis MN, USA) that allows for cauterization of larger areas of tissue. A bipolar set of electrodes is used with saline that is sprayed between them allowing for a deep and wide area of cautery and hemostasis. This is a helpful instrument especially when there is a large area of blood oozing from debrided tissue that has exposed muscle fibers.

pocket. The pocket may then be closed primarily with sutures. Various closure techniques are described including multiple layers with absorbable suture and single interrupted closure with large nonabsorbable monofilament suture such as #1 or #2 nylon or polypropylene. The patient is then placed on some period of targeted antibiotic therapy as noted earlier.

Again, there have been occasional case reports and small series (not to be confused with prospective randomized studies!) of nonrecurrence of infection using this technique. It must be stressed that these success stories are not common and are not always reproducible. The natural course of pocket revision is most often resurgence of the infection at some time, usually weeks to months following the intervention. Virtually every valid series that has looked at antibiotics with or without debridement has shown an unacceptably high rate of infection recurrence.[3]

POCKET RELOCATION

Another option in association with debridement and sterilization is that of pocket relocation. As opposed to the debridement methodology noted earlier, where the device is placed back into the original implant site, this approach follows the debridement and sterilization with placement of the device at a new anatomic site deeper or adjacent to the original site. This is not to be confused with placement of a new system on the contralateral side.[10,14–16]

Once the device is removed from the infected area and the process noted in the debridement section earlier has been completed, a new pocket is then formed is a fresh area, either adjacent to the old implant site (eg, medial or lateral to the original pocket) or in a deeper tissue plane such as the subpectoral space. If the leads are long enough, the device may be moved to a midaxillary position or some area lateral to the original pocket.

Placement of the device into a submuscular area may be an option, especially when the patient is thin. To perform this type of placement, the fibers of the pectoralis major muscle are spread, and the space between the pectoralis major and pectoralis minor fibers is identified. It is also possible to dissect to the back of the pectoralis minor fibers to access the area of the posterior pectoralis fascia; however, the device will sit on top of the ribs and may be more uncomfortable for the patient. There may also be an issue of a large "potential space" in the latter area that could carry an infection along that tissue plane.

Again, because the system is contaminated, chronic antibiotic therapy is then often used to suppress regrowth of the causative microbes. The challenge with this approach is the possibility of new abscess formation at the new location. This may be especially problematic when the new site is very deep in the subpectoral tissue plane.

CHRONIC OPEN DRAINAGE

Some situations exist that may result in an opening over the device that drains chronically, a chronic draining sinus leading to the device pocket, or exposed lead ends that are infected and have eroded through the skin. For example, a patient may have an epicardial lead system associated with an abdominal wall device implant. In the case where the device pocket has been infected, with subsequent removal of the device and cutting of the leads, it is not uncommon for a chronic draining sinus to develop where the leads were cut. Lead erosion at that site may also occur, as well as tracking of the infection along the leads to the intrathoracic space.

When full surgical removal, debridement, or relocation of a system or of the exposed lead portion is not possible, it may be necessary for the patient to live with chronic drainage. If the lead ends are exposed, they may be trimmed back, and the surrounding tissue debrided. This can then be managed with local treatment along with daily bandage changes over the site or even with the use of a small ostomy bag over the area to contain the drainage. The same process is used for a draining sinus that leads to the device pocket. For an infection that has tracked to the intrathoracic space, the use of an Eloesser flap to create a path for chronic drainage has been described.[17] As long as the site remains open and draining, the possibility of systemic infection is reduced. Unfortunately, when foreign material remains present in the tract or pocket, complete cure is not likely using this methodology.

CLOSED POCKET IRRIGATION

An interesting option to attempt a cure is that of closed pocket irrigation.[8,12–15,18–20] This was originally described in the 1980s and several iterations have been proposed in case reports and a few small series. The basic procedure is the same. The pocket is managed as described earlier in the debridement section, assuring that a significant enlargement of the pocket is made. Before primary closure of the incision, one tube is placed through a healthy part of the skin superior to the incision, and one similarly at the base of the pocket. An antibiotic solution is infused into the pocket via one tube, and the effluent is then drained from the second tube (**Fig. 4**).

The major differences described in this approach relate to the type of solution infused and the duration of treatment. Different antibiotics used alone, in combinations, and even with the addition the wetting agent tyloxapol have been described. Various durations of therapy are described, with 4 to 5 days being most common. The irrigation is then stopped, and the drains are removed 24 hours later. The exact duration for which the irrigation should proceed has not been studied, and thus an empirical approach has been used. Success rates for this approach range from 80% to 100%. Although this technique has been shown to have some promise, it has not been studied in any large randomized clinical trial.

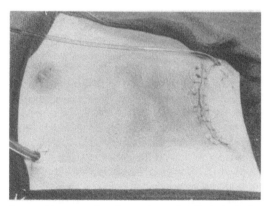

Fig. 4. Photograph of a salvaged infected device pocket that was debrided and closed primarily with a tube for continuous infusion of antibiotic from above and a second tube for drainage from below. Antibiotic is typically infused for up to a week after which the tubes are removed. (*From* Hurst LN, Evans HB, Windle B, et al. The salvage of infected cardiac pacemaker pockets using a closed irrigation system. Pacing ClinElectrophysiol 1986;9(6 Pt 1):790; with permission.)

VACUUM-ASSISTED WOUND CLOSURE THERAPY

Recently, the use of continuous vacuum applied to an infected cavity has been shown to accelerate the healing process.[21] The typical use of this therapy is to address the pocket after the device and lead system have been completely removed and the pocket debrided. However, it has also been reported as a method to effect wound healing and cure without removal of the device and lead system.[22,23] Application of vacuum therapy directly over an open eroded/infected pocket and use of vacuum-assisted wound closure therapy over a pocket that has been debrided with the device placed back into it have been described.

LEAD ABANDONMENT

As noted, it is preferable to remove all prosthetic material from an infected area whenever possible. However, there are some situations when removal of the lead system may be too difficult or dangerous. This may be the case when leads are old and calcified into the venous system, the leads are so large that they cannot be extracted with the current transvenous extraction sheaths that are available, or when leads have been placed on the epicardial surface of the heart. Epicardial leads pose a unique problem in that there are really no transvenous or minimally invasive techniques that can be practically or easily applied to remove them. The leads are tunneled from the epicardial space to a device pocket either in the chest or abdominal wall area. In recent times, this is frequently done for patients who require an epicardial left ventricular lead for cardiac resynchronization therapy when the transvenous approach was not possible. Although somewhat similar to the situation described earlier in the section on chronic drainage, the course of the lead in this case may be quite different, even traversing through the pleural space. Although there are no series to support the technique described here, it has been used successfully several times.

After the infected pocket is debrided and cleansed, and the epicardial lead has been dissected free from the underlying tissues, the lead is pulled on and clamped at the entry site to the chest. The lead is then scrubbed with an antiseptic solution as described earlier. The insulation is circumcised about 1 cm from where it is clamped at the tissue entrance, and the conductor is pulled on while the insulation close to the clamp is pushed toward the clamp. The conductor is then cut, and the remnant is allowed to retract into the insulation close to the clamp. It is then scrubbed again with an antiseptic solution, wiped dry, and silicone medical adhesive is applied to the insulation opening, attempting to infuse adhesive into the open end to seal it. Once this has had some time to set, the clamp is released, and the end of the wire retracts into the chest wall. The area is irrigated again, and the pocket is managed using one of the methods noted earlier. All other foreign materials are now removed, and then the pocket is treated as any other infected pocket for which total device extraction has been achieved. The patient is then treated with targeted antibiotic therapy for 4 to 6 weeks. Using this technique, the authors have not had any recurrences or sequelae related to the cut and retained lead fragment.

It should be noted that in the case of transvenous leads, the "cut and run" method just noted is not recommended. Cutting a retained intravascular lead that is infected frequently results in a persistent bacteremia. If the lead is now not able to be reached from the implant site, transvenous extraction is much more challenging. One may use a femoral approach, or possibly an internal jugular approach, to snare and remove the remaining part of the lead. However, if significant fibrosis is present in the subclavicular area or along the course of the subclavian or innominate vein, then snare retrieval from an alternate site may very difficult or impossible. If the lead system cannot be removed, a full debridement and sterilization approach as noted earlier may occasionally be successful. Cleaning, cutting, sealing, and abandoning the leads in the absence of a pulse generator may occasionally prove to be successful using the same techniques as described for salvage with the entire system in place.

If lead ends that have been abandoned erode through the skin, a unique approach has been described using fibroblastic growth factor to accelerate and promote healing.[4] The growth factor is applied directly to the open wound on a daily basis with dressing changes and cleansing. The intent of the therapy is to enhance growth of tissue and closure of the pocket. Although this is an intriguing concept, it has only been described as a case report.

ANTIMICROBIAL ENVELOPE

An antimicrobial envelope has been available for several years. The first iteration involved the application of 2 antibiotics (rifampin and minocycline) to a polypropylene mesh. Although retrospective studies showed that there was likely some benefit to using this device, there was concern regarding the nonabsorbable nature of the mesh envelope after the antibiotic elution period was complete.

More recently, the introduction of a bioabsorbable version of this envelope has resulted in more widespread acceptance. The envelope is only approved for prophylaxis of infection when one does not exist. Even so, some have used this after wound debridement to hopefully add a high concentration of anti-Staphylococcal therapy. It has also been used after the pocket has been contaminated from a penetrating injury and simple erosion of a portion of a lead.[9,11] It should be cautioned that placing this type of envelope in a grossly infected pocket is not advised and is not likely to result in a cure or even suppression of an abscessed pocket without some other form of intervention as noted earlier.

SUMMARY

The preferred management for patients with CIED infection is complete removal of the entire system. This has been shown to provide the best outcomes, resolving the infection in nearly all cases. For those patients who are too ill, too frail, lack access to transvenous extraction, or have other reasons for not having a total system extraction, there are other options. None of the nonextraction methods are guaranteed; however, in selected cases they provide a real option for palliation, chronic suppression, and in some cases a cure for CIED-related infection. Working with a team of invested, informed consultants is the best way to achieve optimal results for each patient.

REFERENCES

1. Sekiguchi Y. Conservative therapy for the management of cardiac implantable electronic device infection. JArrhythm 2016;12:293–6.
2. Molina EJ. Undertreatment and overtreatment of patients with infected antiarrhythmic implantable devices. Ann ThoracSurg 1997;63:504–9, 3 groups. Group 1(12) Relocation with IV atb (all failed), Group 2(19) removal and 10 days ATB, Group 3(7) 6 wksatb. All 1 failed. The others all successful.
3. Byrd CL. Managing device related complications and transvenous lead extraction in cardiac pacing, defibrillation and resynchronization therapy. In: Ellenbogen KA, Kay GN, Lau CP, et al, editors. Clinical cardiac pacing, defibrillation and resynchronization therapy. Philadelphia: Saunders Elsevier; 2007. p. 855–930, 69 patients 45% success at one year.
4. Fukata M, Arita T, Kadota H, et al. Successful management of wound dehiscence after implantation of a subcutaneous implantable cardioverter-defibrillator without device removal. HeartRhythm Case Rep 2017;3:415–7.

5. Turkisher V, Priel I, Dan M. Successful management of an infected implantable cardioverter defibrillator with oral antibiotics without removal of the device. Pacing ClinElectrophysiol 1997;20:2268–70.

6. Weiner J, Goldberger JJ. Pocket salvage in patients with infected device pocket and limited vascular access: a viable last resort? Pacing ClinElectrophysiol 2011;34:e11–3.

7. Kolker AR, Redstone JS, Tutela JP. Salvage of exposed implantable cardiac electrical devices and lead systems with pocket change and local flap coverage. Ann PlastSurg 2007;59:26–30.

8. Taylor RL, Cohen DJ, Widman LE, et al. Infection of an implantable cardioverter defibrillator: management without removal of the device in selected cases. Pacing ClinElectrophysiol 1990;13:1352–5.

9. Dolacky SD, Wehber AA, Wortham DC, et al. Nailedit: conservative management of penetrating injury and potential infection of a cardiovascular implantable electronic device. Pacing ClinElectrophysiol 2016;39:1412–4. Use of TyRx, pocket revision and irrigation with vancomycin.

10. Knepp EK, Chopra K, Zahiri HR, et al. An effective technique for salvage of cardiac-related devices. Eplasty 2012;12(e8):68–75.

11. Schaller RD, Cooper JC. Salvage of focally infected implantable cardioverter-defibrillator system by in situ hardware sterilization. HeartRhythm Case Rep 2017;3(9):431–5.

12. Glikson M. Conservative treatment of pacemaker pocket infection: is it a viable option? Europace 2013;15:474–5.

13. Lopez JA. Conservative management of infected pacemaker and implantable defibrillator sites with a closed antimicrobial irrigation system. Europace 2013;15:541–5.

14. Hurst LN, Evans EB, Windle B, et al. The salvage of infected cardiac pacemaker pockets using a closed irrigation system. Pacing ClinElectrophysiol 1986; 9(1):785–92.

15. Keeley AJ, Hammersley D, Dissanayake M. Successful conservative management of a permanent pacemaker pocket infection: a less invasive approach. BMJ Case Rep 2017. https://doi.org/10.1136/bcr-2017-220258.

16. Har-Shai Y, Amikam S, Ramon Y, et al. The management of exposed cardiac pacemaker pulse generator and electrode using restricted local surgical interventions; subcapsular relocation and vertical-to-horizontal bow transposition techniques. Br J PlastSurg 1990;43:307–11.

17. Schubmehl HB, Sun HH, Donington JS, et al. An old solution for a new problem: Eloesser Flap management of infect defibrillator patches. Ann ThoracSurg 2017;103:e497–8.

18. Golden GT, Lovett WL, Harrah JD, et al. The treatment of extruded and infected permanent cardiac pulse generators: application of a technique of closed irrigation. Surgery 1973;74:575–9.

19. Furman RW, Hiller AJ, Playforth RH, et al. Infected permanent cardiac pacemaker: management without removal. Ann ThoracSurg 1972;14:54, 5 patients treated with closed irrigation with neomycin, bacitracin and polmyxin.

20. Lee JH, Geha AS, Rattehalli NM, et al. Salvage of infected ICDs: management without removal. Pacing ClinElectrophysiol 1996;19(1):437–42.

21. Gabriel A, Shores J, Bernstein B, et al. A clinical review of infected wound treatment with vacuum assisted closure (V.A.C.) therapy: experience and case series. IntWound J 2009;6:1–25.

22. Poller WC, Schwerg M, Melzer C. Therapy of cardiac device pocket infections with vacuum-assisted wound closure – long term follow-up. Pacing ClinElectrophysiol 2012;35:1217–21.

23. Satsu T, Onoe M. Vacuum-assisted wound closure for pacemaker infection. Pacing ClinElectrophysiol 2010;33:426–30.

Printed and bound by CPI Group (UK) Ltd, Croydon, CR0 4YY

03/10/2024

01040304-0017